ACQUIRING
OPTIMAL
HEALTH

ACQUIRING OPTIMAL HEALTH

Gary Price Todd, M.D.

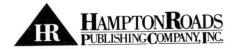

HAMPTON**ROADS**
PUBLISHING COMPANY, INC.

Cover design by Patrick Smith

For information write:

Hampton Roads Publishing Company, Inc.
891 Norfolk Square
Norfolk, VA 23502

Or call: (804)459-2453
FAX: (804)455-8907

If you are unable to order this book from your local
bookseller, you may order directly from the publisher.
Quantity discounts for organizations are available.
Call 1-800-766-8009, toll-free.

ISBN 1-878901-92-3

Printed on acid-free paper in the United States of America

Table of Contents

Foreword

If the term "optimum health" is a phrase frequently bandied about in the halls of medical schools and hospitals, by the medical profession, it has totally escaped my notice in the forty-odd years I have practiced as an internist/cardiologist in the states of Tennessee and Florida; yet such is the underlying theme of Gary Price Todd's present book—*Acquiring Optimal Health*. Since, objectively viewed, readers of this book are likely to be a responsible and elite group, they will be attracted to this concept of optimalness much like a ship floundering at sea to a beacon. For what intelligent layman, no matter how diligently he pursues a working knowledge of nutrition, does not often flounder on the sea of medical nutrition with its conflicting points of view? Only a person possessing a broad knowledge of biochemistry backed by years of clinical observation and experience can write with the authority that Dr. Todd does and produce the results documented here.

I have particular admiration for Dr. Todd's preventive work, because, bluntly put, he has striven to make his own surgical interventions unnecessary as much as possible. At the turn of the century Sir William Osler, an internist, proudly described medicine as "the only profession that strives unceasingly to put itself out of business." Whatever happened to that one? Todd has few peers in this reducing of the need for medical services, alas.

In closing, I might mention that Dr. Todd has personally dealt with a life-threatening illness and has done so successfully. In no small part was this happy outcome accomplished by his practicing upon himself what he preaches to the rest of us.

There is a strong religious undercurrent in these pages and we can do no better than follow the timeless advice of Todd's acknowledged Master Healer in evaluating Todd's or anyone else's teachings: "By Their Fruits Ye Shall Know Them."

Dan C. Roehm, M.D., F.A.C.P.

Preface

I strongly recommend this book to anyone who desires a better quality of life with optimal health and who is also willing to take responsibility for his or her own health. I also recommend this book to physicians who assume a responsibility in guiding their patients toward improved health through nutrition and preventive medicine.

Dr. Todd's first book on nutrition, *Nutrition, Health, and Disease*, provided health-conscious readers with a large volume of facts to show that optimal health can be achieved only with the intake of vitamin and mineral supplements. *Nutrition, Health, and Disease* is now in its fourth edition. Important material in that publication is not covered in this book; so you are advised to read Dr. Todd's prior book.

Acquiring Optimal Health is intended as a guide book or road map for achieving optimal health. The earlier book provides evidence to prove that better health is possible; this book more succinctly tells you how.

Acquiring Optimal Health is the distillation of ten years of Dr. Todd's clinical experience while actively investigating the problems of degenerative, age-associated diseases. Dr. Todd assumes that the reader wishes to enjoy the highest quality of life for whatever years he or she has remaining to live; and he offers practical, workable approaches which can be applied in virtually anyone's life. Dr. Todd's approach is imminently practical and is designed to achieve benefit in the most cost-effective way. Readers who apply these principles to their own lives will be rewarded with better health, increased physical stamina, reduced risk of degenerative diseases and cancer, and a longer, high-quality life span.

Dr. Todd correctly points out that the hysteria over cholesterol is largely misinformed and suggests a sensible approach to lowering cholesterol levels without expensive and potentially dangerous drugs. Beneficial high-density lipoprotein cholesterol is not an enemy. Measurements of total blood cholesterol have little meaning if the beneficial form is present in adequate amounts. In its correct form, cholesterol is an essential nutrient necessary for life, used by the body to defend itself against free radicals.

For those who already suffer from hardening of arteries, even in the presence of elevated, harmful, low-density lipoprotein cholesterol, Dr. Todd intelligently explains how chelation therapy can be a much safer, much less expensive, and more effective option than bypass surgery.

Dr. Todd is primarily an ophthalmologist, but in the process of developing techniques for restoring and preserving vision in patients afflicted with macular degeneration, cataracts, diabetic retinopathy, and other eye diseases, he discovered that it was also necessary to improve the overall physical and metabolic health to obtain and maintain improved vision. Dr. Todd therefore became skilled in restoring general health to the entire body. This book results from his extensive experience.

Elmer M. Cranton, M.D.

Dr. Cranton is a graduate of Harvard Medical School. He is co-author of Bypassing Bypass, *the best-selling book on chelation therapy as an alternative to coronary bypass surgery. He has served as chief-of-staff at a U.S. Public Health Service hospital and is currently engaged in clinical preventive medicine, including chelation and hyperbaric oxygen therapy, in Trout Dale, Virginia.*

1
Introduction

This book is written to give you reasonable guidelines for achieving optimal health. Optimal health is other than being in merely "good" health; *good health* is generally taken to mean that you are not actually sick, whereas *optimal health* means that you are as healthy as you possibly could be. There is ample scientific evidence that with optimal health human beings should live between 100 and 120 years, as a few of us do already. Indeed, this is the Biblical promise dating back at least 5000 years. (For those who might be interested, the promise is found in Genesis 6:3 and Isaiah 65:20-22.)

It is not the purpose of this book to cover what is thoroughly covered in my book *Nutrition, Health, and Disease*, now in its fourth edition and sixth printing. *Nutrition, Health, and Disease* deals primarily with the impact of and need for good nutrition for optimal health. In that book there is great detail of information which will help the responsible reader understand why nutrition is important to good health and why good health is impossible without good nutrition. The purpose of this book is more to tie all the loose ends together, the strings of exercise, diet, lifestyle, pollution, and nutritional supplements. Whereas *Nutrition, Health, and Disease* is intended to almost overwhelm the reader with facts to bring him to the decision that something should be done to improve his health, the purpose of this book is to tell the reader how to do it.

From time to time in this book I mention a source for products recommended. One of these sources is Bio-Zoe,

Inc., an information-sharing network created to make available to its members high-quality information and products aimed at achieving good health. Bio-Zoe may be contacted at P.O. Box 49, Waynesville, NC 28786-0049 (800-426-7581 or 704-452-0472).

Optimal health is a lifelong pursuit. Those who wait until later in life to seek optimal health will find that it will be harder to achieve, and the benefits will not be so great. Most of us enjoy good health while we are young, but during the young adult years, as we become busier and busier with our work and social life, we tend to allow our health to deteriorate and simply borrow from our health to maintain the hectic pace. This is very much like a person who moves money out of his savings account to live on and does not replenish the savings account. Eventually, both approaches will end up in bankruptcy—either financially or in life.

Therefore, you should begin working toward optimal health while you still have your good health. It is far easier to achieve optimal health and to keep it while you are young than it is to wait until your health has deteriorated to the point that you are having significant life-threatening diseases, then attempt to recover your health after having lost it. However, it *is possible* to recover health even in old age. One elderly citizen, now in his late seventies, runs the marathon race annually. Yet he never ran at all before his sixty-fifth birthday when he saw that his health was deteriorating and decided to do something about it.

When we are young, we get out and play hard or work hard and get sore. We realize that we're sore because we are out of condition, and then work hard to get ourselves back into physical shape. When we are old, we get out and work hard and play hard and get sore. But this time we tend to think that the aches and pains are due to old age, not due to simply being out of shape, and we make the unwise decision not to work so hard next time. Thus we age and grow feeble not because of years, but rather because of attitude and lack of knowledge. Professional athletes have the saying "No pain, no gain." This is very true. One cannot generally gain physical strength without some soreness and aching.

Optimal health requires also that we be careful what we put into our bodies, especially today since so many toxic substances are in the air, in the water, and in our food supply. However, optimal health also includes keeping poisonous thoughts out of the mind. What goes on in your mind is every bit as important to your physical health as what goes on in your body, what you eat, and what you drink. The portals of the mind are the eyes and ears. The wise person will be very careful what he sees and what he hears, lest he pollute his mind and fill himself with thoughts that lead to poor health.

In a recent study of one thousand consecutive patients tested for mineral levels, more than 99 percent were deficient in one or more minerals. Specifically, the percent of individuals deficient in various minerals was:

Mineral	Percent deficient
Magnesium	79%
Zinc	94%
Copper	77%
Chromium	99%
Selenium	96%
Manganese	96%

In addition to these deficiencies in essential minerals, 14.4% had significant levels of toxic metals, lead, mercury, and cadmium. (Aluminum, although toxic, was not tallied.) Any amount of lead, mercury, or cadmium is harmful: there is no such thing as totally safe levels of these industrial poisons. Therefore, it should be of interest that measurable levels were found as follows:

Lead	23%
Mercury	18%
Cadmium	45%

Heavy metals are toxic due to their ability to attach themselves to enzymes and proteins, making the enzymes and proteins ineffective. For all practical purposes, each atom of lead, mercury, or cadmium results in one enzyme molecule inactivated. Therefore, any amount of these metals is toxic, and there is no absolutely safe level. As you can see from the list above, exposure to these toxins is almost universal.

Lead seems to affect the central nervous system most and manifests as lowered mental ability, hostility, fits of anger, and an inability to concentrate. If that sounds like a description of inner-city children, then you understand why this problem is not just academic. Most of the lead exposure comes from lead-based paints and leaded gasoline.

Mercury attacks the thyroid gland and also the brain. The phrase "mad as a hatter" derived from the insanity common among hatters who used mercury to produce felt. The two most common sources of mercury are dental amalgams and predator fish: salmon, swordfish, and tuna. Two servings per week of these fish will result in measurable levels of mercury in the hair. Cadmium seems most toxic to the kidneys and can result in hypertension. Glaucoma resistant to therapy seems to be associated with elevated cadmium levels. The usual source of cadmium is automobile tires and galvanized plumbing.

Aluminum, also toxic, is common in most foods. Aluminum buildup in the body seems to be the result of increased permeability (leakiness) of cell membranes, due in turn to hydrogenated fats (margarine and hydrogenated vegetable shortenings) or simply free-radical damage. Aluminum leaves the body quickly once margarine is eliminated from the diet.

Every function of your body requires enzymes. All enzymes have associated with them one or more of the mineral trace elements, either as part of the molecule as in insulin and hemoglobin, or associated with the enzyme as magnesium is in many cases. Without adequate levels of the essential trace minerals, these enzyme systems go begging, and your health is less than optimal.

One key to optimal health, then, is to bring your trace minerals up to optimal levels, and to rid the body of poisonous substances such as lead, mercury, cadmium, and hydrogenated fats. This will be discussed in greater detail later in this book.

2
Exercise and Lifestyle

There is an old saying, worthy of repeating, which says, "Use it or lose it!" This is extremely true in the case of the body and mind. In order to maintain a certain level of physical strength, you must sustain that level of exercise at least fifteen minutes per session, at least three days per week. If you do that you will maintain your present level of physical conditioning. If you wish to increase your level of physical conditioning, you need to increase the frequency that you do this (up to six days per week), and perhaps increase the time to twenty or thirty minutes per session. The exercise should be strenuous enough to work up a sweat, and specifically strenuous enough to raise the heartbeat to a fairly fast pace. Most authorities believe that you should raise the heartbeat to 180 beats per minute minus your age. That is, if you are 50 years of age, you should not raise it above 130 (180-50=130). Actually, this guideline does not really apply to a person who is in excellent health and has been there all his life, but it is generally assumed that if you maintain your pulse rate to that level (180 minus age), that you will not risk a heart attack.

Very obviously, a person who is not currently in good physical condition should consult with a physician before attempting strenuous exercise. Generally speaking, if you are able to work several hours without being overly tired, doing such work as mowing the lawn with a push or power mower or doing other similar strenuous work without chest pain or undue aches or pains, then you should be able to sustain a moderate exercise program. If you are not sure, especially if you are over 45 years of age, you should have a general physical, including a cardiogram, before proceeding.

Once you have decided that your physical condition is satisfactory enough to allow a moderate exercise program, then begin exercising slowly and increase your level of exercise at a slow rate. It takes approximately six weeks for the body to grow new blood vessels to supply the additional blood needed by the more active muscles; so give yourself time to adjust. Rome wasn't built in a day, and it is going to take several months for you to reach your top physical condition. Be patient and persistent in your exercise program. Initially, you will require more rest as your muscles are sore, but as your physical condition improves you will require much less sleep. Enough less, in fact, to offset the time you put into your exercise program. In the end you will have more time and also be able to work more efficiently (due to improved health).

Sleep is extremely important to health for both physical and emotional and spiritual reasons. It is during sleep that the body releases growth hormone essential for growth and muscle development. Growth hormone is released only if sufficient amounts of GTF chromium is present. Chromium is lost if you eat a high-sugar meal in the evening, and especially if your iron levels are high. Therefore, do not frequently eat dessert after the evening meal, and do not take supplements with iron unless you know you are iron-deficient. The most reliable blood test to determine iron levels is the serum ferritin level. Ideally, it should be in the range of 40-100 for optimal health. Serum iron levels can be lowered by donating blood regularly or by intravenous vitamin C. Oral vitamin C increases iron absorption fourfold. This is not a reason for not taking oral vitamin C, but a good reason for not taking supplemental vitamin C and iron. The RDA for iron is based on 10-percent absorption of 18 milligrams of iron. If you take the supplemental vitamin C, the RDA for iron should be met with less than 5 milligrams of iron per day, easily supplied by diet.

If you awaken still sleepy and have difficulty getting out of bed, then you probably need more sleep. On the other hand, if you awaken naturally you may as well get out of bed and make yourself useful. An hour's sleep before 10:00P.M. is probably worth several hours after 10:00P.M. Whether we like it or not, our bodies do respond to the rhythm of day and night, and very specifically to light with a full color spectrum (like natural sunlight). The amount of sleep you actually need varies from individual to individual but generally is in the range of four to ten hours daily. Persons in good physical and emotional health (that is, not under a lot of stress) need less sleep than those out of shape. That is why a physical conditioning program saves time rather than taking time, at least once you have achieved good physical conditioning.

Another reason sleep is so important is emotional and spiritual. The mind works out stressful problems while the body is asleep, one reason a person under stress needs more sleep. More importantly, if you are open to communication from God you will find He will communicate frequently through your dreams. I learned as young as age thirteen that I could solve problems quickly by defining the problem concisely before going to bed and sleeping on it. In many cases I awakened the next morning either with the answer or with a way to discover the answer. Sometimes it took much longer to solve a problem. My Dad, an engineer, gave me a problem at age fourteen, the solution of which required some understanding of calculus. I awakened about 3:00A.M. two or three years later with a solution to the problem and went on to win a regional science fair with the results. The thing I had discovered was to define the problem, then turn it over to my subconscious to work on it. When the subconscious solves the problem, it will toss it up to the conscious mind.

M. Scott Peck, M.D., author of *The Road Less Traveled*, states in his book that he is convinced that the unconscious mind of each of us is the same (identical), and that it is the consciousness of God Himself. I believe he is right. Many persons have been astounded at my abilities and productivity, which I consider mediocre and actually below my potential. The secret to my success, however, is my ability to tap into the consciousness of God, the source of all knowledge and wisdom. My book *The Eternal Triangle* covers this dimension thoroughly.

I strongly advise that you take at least four different supplements during your exercise regimen to speed up your physical conditioning and reduce the risk of harm.

First, take coenzyme Q-10, at least 30 milligrams per day continuously, and during the first two or three months take at least 90 milligrams of coenzyme Q-10 per day. Coenzyme Q-10 does store in the body, so a high dose is not necessary forever, but at least 30 milligrams should be maintained on a regular basis. Coenzyme Q-10 is totally non-toxic, but does have several beneficial side effects. It increases muscle strength 56 percent without exercise. It slows aging and perhaps even reverses the aging process. It also improves the body's immune system and reduces the risk of cancer. Very specifically, it strengthens the heart tremendously and reduces the risk of heart attack. A complete discussion is found in my book *Nutrition, Health, and Disease*.

Second, take 125-250 milligrams of n,n dimethylglycine sublingually about ten or twenty minutes prior to heavy exercise. Dimethylglycine (DMG) is an intermediary metabolite which greatly increases the amount of energy expendable without cramping or muscle aches. It does this by increasing the oxygen level in the tissue and also by decreasing lactic acid build-up. DMG has been proven to increase exercise endurance by 56 percent. It also improves the immune system manyfold and has been proven to reduce the duration of colds and influenza when taken during an infection. Keep some handy when you're doing strenuous exercise, because if taken immediately upon onset of chest pain, it can be life-saving. DMG works with magnesium and coenzyme Q-10 in producing adenosine triphosphate, a major element necessary for the production of energy.

Third, since magnesium is always utilized in production of energy, and since magnesium will prevent muscle aches and pains during severe exercise, you should be taking a minimum of 300 milligrams of magnesium aspartate daily during your exercise regimens. Taking some immediately prior to exercising will reduce the risk of muscle soreness. This effect is enhanced if you take 400-1200 I.U. of natural vitamin E prior to exercise.

Fourth, synthesis of muscle requires growth hormone. Growth hormone is released at night under the stimulation of the presence of adequate levels of chromium. Sugar eaten at the evening meal or at night will block the release of human growth hormone. Therefore, eating dessert after supper or eating a high-sugar meal in the evening reduces the benefit of exercise and also increases the level of fat in the body. Watch your diet and take at least 200-400 micrograms of GTF chromium daily while exercising. It would appear to be most effective if taken with the evening meal. For a person who does not have diabetes, 400 tablets of 200-microgram GTF chromium taken over several months will bring the chromium level up into the low normal range, assuming there is a deficiency at the beginning, which most people have. If you are going to take more than 800 tablets of GTF chromium over a period of twelve months or less, then it's highly recommended that you have a hair analysis performed regularly to prevent toxicity. Excess chromium does leave the body fairly readily; so the risk is low. Non-diabetics can utilize any commercial GTF chromium. Diabetics should use the Chromacin™ formula, the only formulation proven effective in reducing insulin requirements in diabetics.

Specific Recommendations for Exercise

Probably the best and most economical exercise program you can use involves nothing more than a brisk walk. All you need to purchase is a pair of high-quality walking shoes designed to absorb the shock of walking. If you have access to a beautiful area in which to walk, walking can be a time of invigoration and peaceful solitude. However, the walk goes faster if you have someone who will walk with you.

The next step up in strenuous exercise is jogging, but jogging produces much more trauma to the body, especially to the knees, hips, and ankles.

Since cartilage requires manganese to be healthy, and since the vast majority of persons tested in my office are deficient in manganese, it is highly recommended that you be on a supplement supplying adequate quantities of manganese before being on a jogging program. Sufficient quantities of manganese would be at least 20 milligrams of chelated manganese per day. For people who have obtained hair analyses and know that they are severely deficient in manganese, it appears that 40 milligrams of manganese per day for one year will bring their manganese up into the low-normal range. Higher doses are safe, but only if you repeat the hair analysis at six-month intervals to make sure that you do not sustain toxic side effects. Besides being essential to cartilage, manganese is necessary for neutralizing free radicals (discussed later) and also for maintaining the discs between the vertebrae. For that reason, low back pain is one symptom of manganese deficiency.

Persons who exercise vigorously for prolonged periods of time develop a "second wind," at which time they seem to be able to run without further discomfort. This resurgence of energy occurs because the brain releases endorphins in response to the stress, and these endorphins have a morphine-like effect. In fact, continued exposure to endorphins is truly addicting, and persons who run for hours on end are actually feeding their addictions. For the average person, running more than two to five miles per day has no benefit except as preparation for a marathon run.

Whereas walking and jogging require very little expense other than a good pair of shoes, there are three devices which offer mechanically assisted exercise which can be very beneficial and have the advantage of being able to be utilized even during inclement weather. The least expensive of these is a jogging trampoline. Get one at least 36 inches in diameter, since the smaller ones are difficult to use while maintaining your balance. The jogging trampoline has the advantage that it greatly absorbs the shock of running and produces less trauma to the ankles and knees than running outdoors on pavement. Because you must maintain balance on an unstable surface, it exercises more muscles than simply walking or jogging on a hard surface and therefore expends more energy. It has been calculated that for every two minutes of jogging on a jogging trampoline, energy equal to three minutes of jogging on the ground is expended. Therefore, one can achieve good cardiac conditioning more rapidly with a jogging trampoline than one can with regular jogging or walking. The advantage of the jogging trampoline is mainly that it allows vigorous exercise to be performed indoors, in greater safety and comfort.

A second mechanical device is the rowing machine. The rowing machine has the advantage that it exercises all of the major muscles of the body, especially the legs, abdomen, back, shoulders, and arms. Of all the different exercise machines, I believe the rowing machine to be the best. With a rowing machine half of your exercise session is spent facing forward, thereby exercising your back, legs, and biceps, and half the exercises are done facing backwards, exercising the abdomen and triceps.

Other exercise machines which have been used successfully include the treadmill, the stair-climbing simulator, and the ski machine. The first two of these machines have absolutely no advantages over the jogging trampoline, whereas the ski machine gives a fairly thorough whole-body exercise similar to that achieved with the rowing machine. The Schwinn Air Dyne™ is an excellent exercise machine, which, like the Avita™ rowing machine, will still be going strong when your children come into their inheritance.

Unless you have a job that involves manual labor three or more days per week, it is highly advised that you obtain minimally a pair of walking or jogging shoes and to exercise accordingly. All in all, I believe the rowing machine and the jogging trampoline are the most effective and least expensive ways to go if you want a mechanically assisted exercise program.

Strength is achieved by maximally stressing a muscle and holding it at maximum stress for at least ten seconds. (Longer is not needed.) The stress should be repeated at least three times each session. For most muscle groups, this requirement can be met with isometric exercises. For endurance, however, one needs an exercise mild enough that it can be sustained for at least twelve minutes, because the muscle most valuable for endurance is the heart. Dimethylglycine, mentioned earlier, dramatically improves endurance, and coenzyme Q-10 dramatically improves muscle strength. A complete discussion on coenzyme Q-10 and dimethylglycine is found in my book *Nutrition, Health, and Disease.*

Virtually everything you will want to achieve as you seek optimal health is aided by exercise. Exercise produces strength and endurance, which in turn reduces tiredness. Exercise lowers the harmful LDL cholesterol and raises the beneficial HDL cholesterol. Exercise increases the number of blood vessels available to supply blood to vital organs, thereby reducing the risk of heart attack and stroke. And exercise is essential for weight reduction and a trimmer figure.

3
Dietary Principles

Before discussing the specifics of a healthy diet, it is important to take note of some general principles about nutrition. To be healthy, your body needs oxygen from the air, protein, carbohydrates, fiber to help eliminate toxins from the intestines, active (living) enzymes, vitamins, minerals, and pure water.

In the case of air, it should be obvious that clean air is better for our health than is polluted air. However, don't complain about air pollution if you insist on smoking and polluting it for others. It has been calculated that were a tax added to tobacco to pay for the additional medical costs caused by tobacco, the tax would have to be at least $4.00 per pack.

In the case of water, recognize that chlorine is added to municipal water to kill any living organism in the water. If you use chlorinated water to water your garden, yields will be reduced by a third; if you put fish in chlorinated water, they will die. The chlorine is there to keep bacteria and parasites from killing you. There is no doubt in my mind that chlorinated water is poison, and this has been proven beyond question in animal studies. You are not superman; you cannot drink such a poison without risk or harm.

Fluoride has also recently been proven to be a carcinogen, increasing the rate of cancer by as much as 26 percent in municipalities using fluoridated water. Although fluoride was supposedly introduced to prevent tooth decay, there is absolutely no evidence that it even does that when added to the water supply. Those who wish to see the evidence that fluoride is a carcinogen should obtain and read *Fluoride, the Aging Factor* by Dr. John Yiamouyiannis, a doctor of biochemistry. The evidence presented is impeccable and stunning.

Only a bone charcoal filter (manufactured exclusively by Rockland International), a reverse osmosis machine, or a distiller will remove both chlorine and fluoride from water. A plain charcoal filter will not remove fluoride but will remove chlorine. The bone charcoal filter will also substantially reduce water levels of toxic heavy metals such as lead, mercury, and cadmium.

Most persons know the diet should supply protein and carbohydrates. Contrary to the official RDA for protein, adults need only about 45 grams of protein daily because the human body is extremely conservative in recycling amino acids within the body. We need a minimum of 100 grams of carbohydrate per day; otherwise the body will burn protein for energy. Fat is essential for health, but the optimal amount seems to be about 20 to 25 percent of dietary calories, whereas the average American diet gets 45 percent of its calories from fat.

The current fad is to eat only unsaturated fats. Actually, unsaturated fats oxidize very rapidly and are therefore potentially carcinogenic. The oxidation can be slowed by taking extra vitamin E (400-1600 IU) and vitamin C (1000 to 4000 milligrams). Saturated fats, on the other hand, tend to increase cholesterol levels. It appears that as long as the total calories from fat is between 20 and 30 percent, and as long as the percentage of fat that is saturated or un-saturated is at least 10 percent of each, the diet is okay in respect to fats. Since the danger in unsaturated fats is in their becoming oxidized, the prudent person will limit the use of unsaturated fats in cooking, where heat and air react with the hot oil to oxidize it. If you are going to fry, use a saturated fat; it is safer and will taste better.

While on the subject of fats, I wish to point out that the

real health value of unsaturated fats is their essential use by the body to synthesize certain hormone-like substances called prostaglandins. The beneficial prostaglandins serve to prevent stroke and heart attack, as well as retard the spread of cancer. The synthesis of these important compounds requires adequate levels of thyroid hormone, selenium, and vitamin E and is blocked by hydrogenated fats such as margarine. That is why it came as no surprise to me when an article in the *NEJM* on August 12, 1990, proved that hydrogenated fats raise total cholesterol levels and lower the beneficial HDL levels. As I have stated in numerous lectures around North America during the past five years, margarine is too toxic for human consumption. The subjects of cholesterol and hydrogenated fats is covered in my book *Nutrition, Health, and Disease.*

Most of my readers are fully aware of the need for vitamins and minerals in the diet, a subject also thoroughly covered in *Nutrition, Health, and Disease.* Most may be unaware that there are many enzyme systems within the body which operate at higher efficiency if the diet supplies these enzymes. As it turns out, plant protoplasm and animal protoplasm is almost identical, and the RNA and enzymes in plants will pass through the intestinal walls and into the blood without being digested. Furthermore, once in the blood these enzymes function as though they belonged there, as indeed they do. Although the body can make these enzymes, our ability to manufacture enzymes falls off as we age. In any case, taking the enzymes in the diet saves valuable energy for other purposes. Vitamins are simple enzymes which we have lost the ability to synthesize, and that is the only difference between vitamins and enzymes. Most enzymes (vitamins) are destroyed by cooking and time. Therefore, these enzymes are in the highest concentrations in fresh raw vegetables and in the juice. The cellulose cell walls in plants cannot be digested by humans; therefore, the valuable juices and enzymes within these cell walls can be utilized only if the food is thoroughly chewed so that all the cells are broken. If you eat a carrot you will benefit from only about 30 percent of the enzyme nutrition in the carrot, and even then only over a three-hour period. If you use a juicer and separate the juice from the cellulose, then drink the juice, you will benefit from 90 percent of the nutritional value within the juice within twenty minutes!

To give a personal story, I had gout for more than twenty years, with uric acid levels consistently above 10.8. In January 1990, I began eating Sun™ Chlorella (basically dried protoplasm from a type of algae), fifteen tablets per day. Within three weeks my toes were free of pain and of a normal color. I stopped the Chlorella, and three months later my uric acid was still at 7.1 and has subsequently dropped to 6.3. It appears at this time that the protoplasmic enzymes in algae cured my gout by entering my cells and making them function normally! Furthermore, I have confirmed in my person that a mixture of raw carrot juice mixed with either raw Irish potato juice or raw green bean juice is more powerful than insulin in bringing down my blood sugar after a meal. Please note that a machine which merely pulverizes the vegetables rather than separates the juice from the pulp is not satisfactory. I am convinced at this point that drinking two or more glasses of carrot juice daily will result in vastly improved health for most persons. To be effective, the juice must be consumed within minutes of extracting the juice, preferably on an empty stomach. Canned or frozen juice, although delicious, does not supply the same nutrition because the enzymes are largely dead and inactive. A quality juicer can be a lifesaver.

Although fresh juice obtained by a juicer is clearly superior, there are other sources of enzymes and also of trace minerals. Spirulina™, a dried algae from mineral ponds in Mexico, is an excellent source of both trace minerals and enzymes, as is the Sun™ Chlorella, a Japanese product. A strictly vegetable product, also from

Japan (and now also the USA), is Barley Green™, made from dried juice from young barley plants, plus kelp for trace minerals and iodine. There are several similar products on the market, all essentially the juice of young plants dried by a low-temperature vacuum process.

Another excellent commercial product is BioStrath™, composed of lysed yeast. Essentially, the yeast is grown in a trace-element-rich nutrient broth until the yeast cells swell up and burst (lyse), at which time herbs and flavorings are added. It is a Swiss product which definitely works to better the health of those who use it. I have enough experience with several of these products to know that they improve the health of persons whose diet of dead and stale foods has led to poor health. If you are traveling, the commercial products are easier to pack and use than a juicer! I personally use a juicer at home, plus Sun™ Chlorella and Barley Green™ for convenience.

The reader should be aware that with all of these products benefits will be noted within two weeks, but after a few weeks or months you will become accustomed to the greater vitality and will not notice the benefit. At that time a lower maintenance dose can be used for greater economy.

A Safe and Sane Diet

Eliminate, to whatever degree possible, white sugar and white flour products, as well as products to which salt has been added. Read the label; sugar and salt are frequently the first or second ingredients of many processed foods. Highly processed foods have most of the nutritional value removed during processing. That is why they will keep on the grocery shelf: the nutritional value is so low that even the vermin cannot survive on it. *Also eliminate fried foods*, again so far as practical, especially those fried in vegetable oils or vegetable shortening. If you do eat fried foods, fry them in either butter or animal fat, beef suet being ideal. *Vegetable oils for frying should be* *minimized, and then used only once*, since they oxidize very quickly, producing toxic free radicals.

Your diet should include at least one or two fruits per day. Consume as much as possible of your fruit and vegetables raw and unprocessed, eating the peelings whenever practical. Be sure to wash the fruit before consumption to remove pesticide residues. Fruit and vegetables that must be cooked should be cooked minimally by steaming or in a microwave oven.

Fat should be trimmed from meats before cooking. Since the fat in poultry is in the skin, remove the skin before consuming. Hamburger and other ground meat should be purchased as fresh as possible, should be used as soon as practical, and should be purchased in the lowest-fat form available.

Eggs are good nutrition and should not be neglected. Forget the bugaboo that eggs raise your blood cholesterol. Eggs cooked without breaking the yolk sack do not materially raise cholesterol levels, since eggs contain the beneficial HDL form of cholesterol. However, if the yolk is broken during the cooking process the cholesterol is converted into the harmful LDL form. Therefore, eggs scrambled or cooked as an omelet should be avoided.

Vegetable oils are essential: the seed foods indicated below should supply them. Of the nuts providing essential fats, pecans and black walnuts are especially good. However, taking one tablespoon of fresh safflower oil per day is recommended. This may be part of a salad dressing.

Sea salt is preferred over regular table salt. Herbal mixtures are available which enhance flavor without adding sodium. In any case, less sea salt than regular table salt is needed to enhance flavor. Shop carefully, however; much that passes for sea salt is merely mined salt to which minerals have been added.

Avoid margarine and all hydrogenated fats. These fats interfere with the body synthesis of essential prostaglandins and also alter the cells' metabolism. Persons who consume these fats have a remarkably increased risk of cancer and perhaps also an increased risk of stroke or heart attack. Butter is neutral in this regard. A thorough discussion of this topic is found in my book *Nutrition, Health, and Disease*. Two studies published in August 1990 have proven the toxicity of these synthetic fats. Those who read my book *Nutrition, Health, and Disease* have known since 1985 that hydrogenated fats are toxic.

Vegetables and Fruit:

Your diet should supply daily at least two generous servings of dark yellow or dark green vegetables or fruit. Especially good are spinach, broccoli, kale, sweet potatoes, pumpkin, squash, peaches, apricots, cantaloupe, and watermelon. Each of these is an excellent source of beta-carotene, proven to be effective in preventing cancer. Include at least one serving of the cabbage family each day, either raw or cooked. These include cabbage, broccoli, Brussels sprouts, turnips, rutabagas, and cauliflower. Also, frequently include onions and garlic, either raw or cooked. As discussed above, buy a quality juicer to get the maximum benefit from your vegetables.

Seed and Grains:

Basically, eat two servings of seed foods daily. That is, foods that reproduce themselves: beans, corn, peas, peanuts, nuts, sunflower seed, wheat, barley, pumpkin seed, and so forth. Many seeds, such as mung beans and alfalfa, are better sprouted and used with a salad. When you buy your bread, try to select one that has a mixture of several grains. Beans are best cooked as a mixture of bean types, since each one has a slightly different mixture of amino acids, and a mixture is therefore a more complete protein. If you garden, grow soybeans and pick when full and still green. Drop in boiling water to shell. Soybeans freeze well and taste a lot like a cross between boiled peanuts and lima beans: a real taste treat for those of us of Southern ancestry.

Meat:

Eat at least one serving of meat a day to get your protein most efficiently. However, millions of vegetarians have proven that humans have no intrinsic need to eat meat and may be healthier without it. I have no objection to red meat, but do recommend that the fat be trimmed. Hamburger should be purchased as lean as possible and as fresh as possible and should be cooked as soon as possible. Liver should be eaten at least once weekly to supply valuable vitamin A; if you do not wish to eat liver, then take a cod liver oil capsule daily.

Fish, especially, should be eaten two or three times per week. It is best eaten baked or broiled, rather than fried, to reduce fat. Fish grill very well on a grill just as one might grill hamburgers. Certain fish provide an essential fatty acid which appears to reduce the risk of heart disease. These include tuna, salmon, trout, sardines, herring, cod, haddock, and mackerel. Note, however, that tuna, salmon, and swordfish also contain a lot of mercury thanks to our propensity to poison the entire planet. More than one serving of these three fish per week will definitely increase your mercury loads. Therefore, go easy on eating them.

Since poultry has its fat in the skin, which can be easily removed, poultry is an excellent source of protein without fat. Be sure to trim off the skin before consuming. Precook chicken in a pressure cooker for eight minutes, batter, and brown in butter for fried chicken that is out of this world and safer than standard fried chicken.

Dairy Products:

I cannot strongly endorse homogenized milk, since there is evidence that the small fat particles in homogenized milk may pass through the intestine into the bloodstream without digestion, possibly producing allergic reactions. I can support the use of raw whole milk which has not been homogenized or pasteurized, assuming the cows can be certified free of tuberculosis and bovine leukemia virus. Without that certification, raw milk is not worth the risk. Skim milk or powdered milk would be superior to homogenized or whole milk. Low-fat acidophilus milk appears to be superior to regular homogenized milk. Better yet would be raw, unpasteurized, non-homogenized milk from a certified farm. I do not think that milk used in cooking has the same problem as homogenized milk consumed as a beverage. Ideal dairy products include yogurt, cottage cheese, and regular cheese. The hard cheeses have less fat and more protein. I would recommend one or two servings daily. Goat's milk is better tolerated by humans than is cow's milk.

Butter is far superior to margarine, which should be avoided along with all hydrogenated fats. Raw creamery butter as found in a health food store has that superior taste those of us raised on a farm remember. Your taste buds have not gone stale: raw butter still tastes as good as it always did. It costs a lot more, but is worth a lot more. Try it: you owe it to yourself to go first class at least once.

Enzymes:

In addition to proteins, fats, carbohydrates, vitamins, and minerals, there is a sixth class of nutrient, namely living enzymes, mentioned above. It has now been proven that active enzymes, when ingested, do enter the blood stream and do benefit the human body. This is the mechanism of action of such prescription drugs as thyroid hormone, estrogens, and progesterones. Unfortunately, living enzymes which are available in all living plant and animal cells are destroyed during cooking. They also begin the process of dying at the time of harvesting or the death of the animal. Currently, it appears that the safest way to get these enzymes into the body is by consuming fresh juice extracted from vegetables using a juicer. I recommend one glass of fresh carrot juice, consumed on an empty stomach, twice daily.

4

Pure Water

Not only should you be careful to ingest only pure and quality foods, but you should also make sure your water is pure and wholesome. Water is often neglected as a nutrient. Ideally, your water should be either pure spring or well water, assuming that it has not been contaminated with industrial waste. If this is not available, then by all means obtain distilled or bottled water. Commercially processed water contains alum, chlorine, and fluoride, all of which are toxic.

Minerals

Only about twelve essential minerals are available in tablet form. However, the human body requires fifty-two minerals, and these must be supplied by the food but generally are not. It is strongly urged that you add ¼ to ½ ounce of Earth Food™, Mineral Toddy™, or similar colloidal minerals per gallon of drinking water and drink this as your water. This will supply the remaining forty essential trace minerals necessary for health. There is simply no economical way to get these trace minerals today except through the supplementation with a colloidal mineral supplement. (See Chapter 5)

By federal and state law, municipal water supplies are required to add chlorine to kill bacteria and protozoa, and in many cases alum to precipitate solids in the water. Whereas this treatment does prevent the water supplies from transmitting deadly communicable diseases, the poison remains in the water for public consumption. Even though the EPA has already issued a memorandum saying that taking a single shower using municipal chlorinated water will raise the household chlorinated hydrocarbon concentration to beyond acceptable levels, and research has proven that drinking chlorinated water is a cause of atherosclerosis, neither the federal nor state governments have addressed this problem. Now it turns out additionally that many water supplies contain unacceptable levels of lead, due in large measure to the use of solder in copper plumbing.

Fluoride is added to most municipal water supplies in an effort to prevent dental cavities. However, evidence is mounting that fluoride does not prevent dental cavities; and worse, fluoride is actually a carcinogen, increasing the risk of cancer by as much as 28 percent in municipalities which have used fluoride for many years. Several European nations have already banned fluoridation of water supplies. (If you do use distilled water or spring water, realize that it will not contain sufficient fluoride to prevent dental cavities, if such a benefit can be proven to exist. Fluoride in low doses may be beneficial, whereas high doses of fluoride are toxic. Commercial fluoride mouthwashes and toothpastes are available to protect the teeth. Their use is recommended.)

In addition to these chemicals added by law, trace amounts of PCBs, pesticides, and industrial chemicals have found their way into our water supplies, including well and spring water.

Reverse osmosis units will remove the majority of both types of contaminants. The major disadvantage of such devices is expense and difficulty of maintenance. Usual distillation units will remove all of the heavy metals but will leave trace amounts of chlorine and volatile hydrocarbons. Activated charcoal filters are very effective in removing hydrocarbon components and chlorine, but do very little to remove heavy metals. Some distillation units put a charcoal filter before and after the distillation process, thereby making this distillation combination one of the most effective methods available for purifying water.

A fourth option now is available. Bone charcoal is currently used in food processing, primarily sugar refining, and for the pharmaceutical industry. Bone charcoal is manufactured from the bones of cattle, fired at high temperatures to produce an activated charcoal which has a large amount of calcium hydroxyapatite crystals. The activated charcoal surface acts as any activated charcoal in removing organic chemicals such as chlorine, pesticides, and PCBs. The calcium, being a relatively active element, will replace ions of lead, cadmium, mercury, iron, aluminum, copper, and other heavier metals plus fluoride in the water. The quantity of heavy ions that is replaced is proportional to the contact time (that is, the flow rate of water). Although removal of toxic heavy metals in this manner can never be total, tests have shown well over 90-percent reduction in many situations. In addition to reducing toxic heavy metals, the passage of calcium into solution reduces the acidity of water; therefore, these units can be beneficial in treating water supplies which are acid.

The Rockland USA Corporation has an exclusive contract with a British manufacturer of Brimac 216™ bone charcoal to use their charcoal for water filters. This is the same bone charcoal used for purifying drugs and white sugar. Rockland makes units which are designed for use at a sink and may be mounted either temporarily on the top of a counter with connections to the faucet, or under the counter with connections simultaneously to an ice maker and a water dispenser. The water dispenser unit is optional at extra cost. This device will purify water at approximately one-half gallon per minute for an average 3,000 gallons. Unlike other units currently on the market, the filter can and should be backwashed, and the bone charcoal can be replaced at substantial savings. This is the only personal water purifier available on the market today which uses bone charcoal, and will be the only one for some time in the future due to contract. Rockland USA also produces units capable of handling up to 160 gallons per minute. Ideally, since you should prefer to bathe in chlorine-free water, a whole-house unit should be considered. However, the Rockland personal model has the distinct advantage of being able to purify drinking and cooking water without great expense. (For a cost of $199 you can purify the equivalent of over $3000 in bottled water.) The unique features of the Rockland USA filter are: 1) use of bone charcoal which reduces or removes heavy metals and organic toxins; 2) replaceable bone charcoal; 3) ability to be used on counter top, under counter, and simultaneously for purification of ice water, and 4) ability to be backwashed and sterilized.

In view of the fact that all municipal water supplies have toxic levels of chlorine and other chemicals added during the processing of water, and perhaps one-third of the nation's water supplies have toxic levels of heavy metals according to the EPA, *every* family should seriously consider installation of a water purification system in the interest of health. *In short, for your improved health, you should be drinking only spring water, well water, bottled water, or municipal water which has been purified either with a combination distillation/charcoal filter, or with a filter that uses bone charcoal such as the Rockland USA filters.* You may buy the Rockland USA Model 70 directly from Bio-Zoe, Inc. for self-installation. Installation is very simple and can be done by anyone in a matter of minutes. If you desire to put the unit beneath the counter with a spout for drinking water, there is a an optional kit which includes fittings for simultaneous purification of ice water.

5
Vitamin and Mineral Supplements

A few years ago I enlisted the cooperation of a computer firm in California to use their computer which had in its memory the nutritional contents of several thousand different commonly eaten foods. I asked them to help me to devise a one-week diet that met all of the known recommended dietary allowances of vitamins and minerals. Although the three diets they proposed were far better than I eat, and certainly far better than the diet of anyone whom I know, they were all deficient in a minimum of eight different minerals and vitamins. One could change the diet slightly to improve the nutritional supply of one or others of the vitamins and minerals, but in so doing would decrease the amount of another nutrient. Therefore, *I must conclude that it is absolutely impossible to meet all necessary nutritional needs with an unsupplemented diet.*

Based on ten years' clinical experience, I would recommend the following vitamins and minerals be taken daily. All of the vitamins included in this list are part of the Nutri-Plex™ formula developed by me and sold by Bio-Zoe, Inc. The current formula of Nutri-Plex™ is as follows. Four tablets contain:

Vitamin A	10,000 IU
Beta-Carotene	10,000 IU
Vitamin D_3	200 IU
Vitamin E	400 IU
Vitamin C	500 mg

Vitamin B_1	25 mg
Vitamin B_2	10 mg
Vitamin B_6	25 mg
Vitamin B_{12}	25 mcg
Vitamin K_1	60 mcg
Niacin	50 mg
Pantothenic Acid	150 mg
Folic Acid	800 mcg
Biotin	300 mcg
Choline	50 mg
Inositol	50 mg
PABA	50 mg
Citrus bioflavinoids	100 mg
Calcium	200 mg
Magnesium	400 mg
Iodine	150 mcg
Copper	2 mg
Manganese	20 mg
Potassium	50 mg
Zinc	20 mg
Molybdenum	200 mcg
Chromium	200 mcg
Selenium	200 mcg
Vanadium	200 mcg
Boron	2 mg
Coenzyme Q-10	10 mg
MSM Sulphur	100 mg
Silica	40 mg

This formula has been modified several times over the last five years based on clinical experience and may be revised further in the future. However, at this time, this appears to be the best general supplement available today. I intend to keep it that way. A detailed description of why these nutrients are important is the theme of my book *Nutrition, Health, and Disease.*

As we discussed in the previous chapter, the human body, in order to remain healthy, needs approximately fifty-two minerals in order to remain healthy, twelve of which are available in tablet form through either Bio-Zoe, Inc., or the average health foods store. The remaining forty essential elements must be found in your food or taken as a supplement, or you will suffer from less than optimal health. At the present time, the best source of these additional forty elements is a commercial product called Earth Food™. (I receive no commission from my recommending the product and have no direct financial ties with the company. However, I do use the product personally and it is also sold by Bio-Zoe, Inc.)

For a person in good health, I believe that ¼ ounce of Earth Food™ per day is sufficient to maintain optimal health. For persons in more severe mineral deficiency, I recommend up to 3 ounces per day, taken either straight or mixed with fruit juice. An ideal way to take Earth Food™ with very little pain is to mix ¼ to ½ ounce of Earth Food™ with one gallon of distilled water and drink your water from this. This produces an extremely high-quality mineral water which supplies fifty-two trace minerals essential to good health. The reader is referred to the chapter on hair analysis to learn how to determine whether or not minerals are in balance.

Remineralization: The Key to Restored Health

Earth Food™ is an extremely concentrated aqueous solution of pure natural minerals and trace minerals. It is extracted from a natural sedimentary deposit of prehistoric plant origin. Basically, Earth Food™ contains the minerals found in prehistoric vegetation 30 million years ago.

During the past two centuries, our nation has been very wasteful in its conservation of soil, so that literally billions of tons of topsoil are being lost each year. Along with this topsoil go the valuable minerals essential to life. In order to keep the crops growing, the farmers are adding back those minerals known to be essential for plant growth, namely calcium, magnesium, potassium, phosphorous, nitrogen, and occasionally also manganese and boron. Whereas plants need only a few minerals for active growth, they will ordinarily assimilate the other trace minerals present in the soil, and we obtain these by eating the plants or the animals which eat the plants. If these minerals are absent or deficient in the soil, as they increasingly are today, then the plants may be healthy but will not adequately supply the proper minerals necessary to sustain healthy life. Any farmer can tell you that this is already a problem with livestock.

Unless you are exceedingly unusual, you are already suffering from reduced health, the direct result of your mineral deficiencies. USDA says that over 98 percent of Americans are mineral-deficient. Of more than 800 consecutive mineral analyses done through my office, over 99 percent showed deficiencies of one or more essential minerals. The minerals found in Earth Food™ are essential for every biologic process that goes on within the body and are therefore essential for life itself. Further information is found in my book *Nutrition, Health, and Disease.*

There are two ways your physician may test for mineral deficiencies, the least expensive being a hair analysis. Blood studies for mineral levels covering a comparable twenty-one minerals would cost over $400. Each type of test has advantages and limitations, but because of cost I prefer the hair analysis with follow-up blood tests when indicated. If you do have a severe deficiency, which is highly likely, you may correct it by taking selected minerals available from your pharmacist or health foods store and be able to restore normal mineral balance within a decade, plus or minus a few years. You can also have the trace minerals given intravenously and restore mineral balance with perhaps twenty infusions given over several months. The cost for re-mineralizing your body in this manner would be about $2500, plus $200 in necessary laboratory tests. Another alternative is the use of Earth Food™. The colloidal nature and high concentration of Earth Food™ makes it an ideal means of correcting mineral deficiencies. Each quart contains over 38,000 milligrams of essential minerals, and its colloidal make-up means that it is better assimilated and less toxic. Since your body will need time to assimilate the minerals present in any food, including Earth Food™, it is recommended that consumption be restricted to 3 ounces daily, taken straight or mixed with fruit juice. A repeat hair analysis should be done annually, and once a satisfactory mineral level is achieved consumption of Earth Food™ should be reduced to about ¼ to 1 ounce daily.

At first glance, Earth Food™ appears to be very expensive; the current price is $100 per gallon. Each quart contains approximately the amount of minerals found in the average diet over nine months, thus a gallon would supply minerals that would take three years to obtain through regular meals. This does not take into consideration that the minerals found in Earth Food™ are far better absorbed than those in tablet form and thus might be expected to achieve faster results.

Some persons may develop diarrhea during the first week of using Earth Food™. This is a natural part of the body detoxifying itself. Unless you feel very ill (other than just being inconvenienced), you should continue use of Earth Food™. An alternative choice would be to temporarily reduce the amount until symptoms subside. This inconvenience is rare and usually lasts only about a week. As with any other food product, an allergic reaction is possible. If you are allergic to Earth Food™ discontinue its use.

Earth Food™ has an interesting side effect due to its colloidal nature and strong negative charge. Several ounces consumed when intoxicated will produce almost instant sobriety. Consumed during a stroke it appears to restore circulation almost immediately. Sprayed on a wound or sunburn it promotes healing and is a mild antibiotic.

Earth Food™ will definitely remove toxic aluminum, lead, cadmium, and mercury from the body when consumed daily over a period of one to two years. The study, done by me, used 3 ounces of Earth Food™ plus 3,000 milligrams of vitamin C daily. Subsequently, the manufacturer has made a product, named Total Toddy™, which combines the ingredients in Earth Food™ with vitamin C and other vitamins and flavorings. Since Earth Food™ has a strong taste, the Total Toddy™ is distinctly more palatable.

There are two products identical to Earth Food™: Mineral Toddy™ and Mystic Minerals™.

6
Hair Analysis

In studies of more than 1000 patients over a two-year period, one in six has proven to have toxic levels of either lead, mercury, or cadmium. A much higher percentage have toxic levels of aluminum, thought by some to be a major cause of Alzheimer's disease. Even more importantly, fully 98 percent of those tested show clinically significant deficiencies in one or more essential trace minerals. The minerals almost universally deficient include chromium, selenium, and manganese. Other common deficiencies include zinc, copper, and magnesium. These minerals are important to a person's health. Selenium, for example, is essential to slow the aging process and also as a preventive of cancer. Zinc is involved in over 370 different enzyme systems of the body including insulin. A deficiency in zinc means that the body cannot have all of the enzymes necessary for good health. Indeed, a deficiency of any mineral means that the body is going begging for those enzymes necessary for good health.

The fastest way to determine your relative levels of minerals is to obtain a hair analysis. The laboratory used by Bio-Zoe, Inc., is accurate and efficient. If the hair analysis is ordered through Bio-Zoe, Inc., it will be analyzed by a computer program written by me. In the alternative, you may send a hair analysis done by another lab and get a computer analysis for a modest fee. This computer program will recommend the proper doses of minerals necessary to bring you back into mineral balance over a two-year period of time. Once you have achieved mineral balance, you will want to repeat the hair analysis at two- to five-year intervals just to check on your toxic mineral exposure. If you or members of your family have not had a hair analysis, I strongly urge you to do so as soon as possible. Please be aware that a permanent, some hair dyes, or anti-dandruff shampoos will change the mineral balance in the hair. The hair analysis is not perfect but is a reliable indicator of the relative amounts of essential trace minerals found in the body.

Most physicians, being ignorant of the advantages of hair analysis, consider the procedure to be fraudulent and quackery. The truth is that for those minerals which are stored in the muscles, skin, and hair, a blood test reveals absolutely nothing. For those minerals, a test of the tissue itself is necessary, and hair is the most readily available and least painful to obtain. Although head hair is preferred, body or pubic hair is satisfactory. Since hair grows slowly, the analysis will represent the average mineral balance in the body over a period of six to eight weeks prior to taking the hair sample.

If your hair analysis indicates significant deficiencies, these can be corrected most quickly and economically by intravenous therapy over a period of two or more months, in ten to twenty intravenous doses. Oral correction of some deficiencies, especially magnesium and selenium, may take several years.

When we provide a computer printout of a hair analysis, we tell the patient that, in general, if he is in excellent overall health, he can safely ignore the printout of the hair analysis and its recommendations and simply take Nutri-Plex™ vitamins twice daily (adult dose). It is our experience that this will fairly rapidly bring minerals into line, with balance being achieved over a period of three to five years. On the other hand, if his health is not optimal and he needs something to be done, then the printout from the enclosed hair analysis sheet should be followed closely.

Kidney function in elderly people may be less than optimal, so they retain a higher percentage of minerals inside their system and thereby can get by with lower doses. If the doses of minerals recommended cause you to retain fluid, then reduce the dose you are taking or increase your consumption of water. Just as too much sodium in the diet will cause water retention, too many minerals in the diet can do the same. However, since kidney function is reduced in the elderly, it is entirely possible that you might be able to get by with a one-third or two-thirds reduction in the recommended dose. However, be aware that the manganese and coenzyme Q-10 generally recommended do improve kidney function. If you are not retaining fluid, then you are not getting too much of minerals, either the ones we recommend or sodium.

For children under fourteen years of age, the dose should be adjusted according to body weight relative to an adult weight of 150 pounds. A child weighing 75 pounds, for example, should take one-half the adult dose.

Calcium is not normally found inside the healthy cell. Therefore, a high level of calcium in your hair indicates a diseased state. It probably is the result of cell membranes being leaky, which in turn can be due to hydrogenated fats (margarine) in the diet or a high level of free-radical activity. If your calcium levels are high, you are strongly urged to get off margarine and hydrogenated fats and take borage seed oil, 1 capsule per day with meals, for at least three months. Another product designed to heal sick cellular membranes is the German supplement Calcium EAP. At this point, it appears that the lower the calcium is in the hair, the healthier you are. Therefore, ignore a low calcium level in the hair, and be thankful. Until recent scientific evidence is confirmed, Bio-Zoe, Inc. will not recommend calcium supplements in excess of about 500 milligrams per day; there is evidence that higher doses of calcium may be detrimental to health.

All of the information in the hair analysis is fed through

a computer program. Interpretation of the data of hair analysis is not simple and must be computed using a computer; otherwise the information coming out is useless. The printout is based on clinical experience with several hundred individuals over many months of time. The equations used are being modified at three-month intervals based on the previous data so that our end results are being continuously improved.

At the present time, *fully one out of six individuals tested has toxic levels of lead, mercury, or cadmium.* Therefore, it strongly behooves all of us to have hair tested at least once in our lives, and if normal to have that repeated at five-year intervals. This test is inexpensive and can literally save your life.

The hair analysis does not test for most of the known essential minerals, largely because these minerals are present in such small amounts as to make detection almost impossible and extremely expensive. The safest course to guarantee adequate amounts of these essential minerals is to use a product such as Mineral Toddy™, described above.

If you prove to have potentially toxic levels of lead, mercury, or cadmium, you will certainly want to get it out. The fastest and most expensive way is through chelation therapy, discussed in the following chapter. If the levels are not extreme, and you're not obviously suffering from the toxic effects of these heavy metal poisons, then taking large doses of vitamin C (which is a mild chelator) plus 1 to 3 ounces of Mineral Toddy™ daily will remove the heavy metals over a period of one to two years. This is effective for lowering aluminum, lead, cadmium, and mercury loads.

A newer product by the same manufacturer, Total Toddy™, combines vitamin C with the ingredients in Mineral Toddy™, plus flavorings.

7
Chelation Therapy

Most of the vitamins and minerals associated with improved resistance to cancer and reduced aging also turn out to be chelates. A chelate is a substance which attaches itself to another molecule, making it soluble. The word itself is Greek for *claw* and graphically portrays what the chelate actually does, grasping and seizing the ion to be chelated.

All life depends upon chelates. Digestion and assimilation of nutrients depend upon chelation; ordinarily insoluble substances are made soluble so that they can pass through the walls of the intestines into the bloodstream. Minerals which have been added to the nutrient broth for yeast become chelated, and therefore are more easily assimilated than non-chelated minerals when used in a supplement. Assuming there is no allergy to yeast products, there are fewer side effects. Some minerals necessary for life are of no benefit unless they are in a chelated form. In fact, some enzymes and vitamins are actually trace-element chelates.

Chelation is the method of action of many of the drugs used today, from antibiotics to pain medications. Chelates are rather specific as to which ion they attract and bind, so there are literally thousands of chelates used daily in medicine and industry. Chelation is absolutely necessary for life and health, both naturally and therapeutically.

The fact that nutritional therapy is effective in restoring health is largely due to chelation by the relatively weak natural chelates, such as vitamin C. Were our diet to have sufficient amounts of these substances, chelation therapy with stronger synthetic substances would not be necessary. Nevertheless, chelation therapy by dietary supplementation is effective, albeit slow.

EDTA is a synthetic amino acid first used in human therapy in 1947. It has a strong affinity for metal ions, and will "drop" one ion if another is available for which it has a higher affinity. The order of affinity, from highest to lowest, is: chromium 2+, iron 3+, mercury 2+, copper 2+, lead 2+, zinc 2+, cadmium 2+, cobalt 2+, aluminum 3+, iron 2+, manganese 2+, calcium 2+, and magnesium 2+. By delivering EDTA as magnesium EDTA, the chelating physician is not only removing toxic metal ions, but also administering magnesium, which is apt to be deficient. Other deficiencies can be corrected in the same way, but obviously if chromium EDTA were administered, only chromium EDTA would be excreted. Except for chromium and zinc, most of the ions for which EDTA has a high affinity are toxic heavy metals, or those which catalyze free-radical reactions. Given intravenously, it will remove those ions by chelation and excretion through the kidneys. It will also remove some beneficial ions, such as zinc and chromium, and these will have to be replaced orally or intravenously. EDTA has been used intravenously safely over six million times in over 400,000 patients in the United States alone. Its success rate in restoring circulation to clogged arteries approaches 82 percent, with less risk, greater effectiveness, and at one-tenth the cost of vascular surgery.

It is uncertain just how chelation works, but there is speculation that EDTA binds excess iron and copper (plus toxic heavy metals), thus preventing much free-radical activity. It appears that it is this inhibition of free-radical activity that allows the body's natural healing processes to repair the damage from free radical pathology. Another interesting discovery is that lactic acid is a chelating agent. Lactic acid is produced during vigorous exercise, and its action as a chelating agent may explain why exercise is so beneficial. Unfortunately, most patients requiring chelation therapy have allowed their physical condition to deteriorate so much that exercise is almost impossible. If you establish a regular exercise program and stick with it, it is likely you can avoid both bypass surgery and chelation. But you will not avoid the need to reduce free-radical damage by use of nutritional therapy.

Is EDTA safe? Go to your pantry, and you will see that you consume EDTA with almost any food you eat. It is added to virtually all processed foods to stabilize them and prevent spoilage. It is also used in shampoos, detergents, water softeners, and an amazingly long list of other products. EDTA is safe. EDTA does not pass readily through the walls of the intestines, so oral consumption is not effective for internal chelation. It is effective, though, in preventing metal ions in food from being absorbed. Used intravenously, it has a therapeutic index far superior to aspirin. (The therapeutic index is a measure of safety.)

EDTA should be used cautiously in persons with renal disease. However, I have polycystic kidney disease and eighteen chelation treatments with EDTA raised my creatinine clearance from 62 (low) to 92 (barely normal). Five years have now passed, and my creatinine clearance has again dropped to 52, so I will soon begin chelation therapy again.

EDTA chelation therapy is usually performed by physicians who themselves resorted to it when their options in life finally ran out. Their successful recoveries have made them a rather enthusiastic group. Unfortunately, these courageous physicians perform this service to others at great personal risk, since organized medicine has generally been against this mode of therapy. This has put the chelation therapists at great risk of legal action and the loss of their licenses to practice medicine, although as physicians they certainly have the right to do what is best for their patients. Health insurance generally will not pay for treatments, which cost about $100 for each of the twenty or more treatments needed. Such costs are a force against the use of this type of therapy.

There are risks if EDTA is infused too fast, but decades of experience have virtually eliminated this risk if the administering physician has followed the proper protocol. [Full information is available from the American College of Advancement in Medicine, 23121 Verdugo Drive, Suite 204, Laguna Hills, CA 92653. Their telephone is (714) 583-7666.] Physicians interested in this mode of therapy are strongly advised to follow the training and treatment protocols and to earn their certificates of qualification. Patients who are interested in chelation therapy are even more strongly advised to seek only the services of chelation physicians certified by this academy. Just as with every profession, medicine has its few bad eggs, and some have gone into production-line chelation. Properly done, chelation takes at least three and a half hours per treatment, and there is no way to shorten that time safely. Some few clinics (chelation mills might be a better name) are pushing infusion rates to the limits of toleration in order to increase profits. It is important that both concerned physicians and patients take an open stand against such practices now before these few charlatans destroy chelation and eliminate its a chance to become an accepted mode of therapy.

Actually, chelation with EDTA has been used by physicians for thirty years. Unlike the current rash of drugs, EDTA is cheap and its patent has long since run out. Its safety record is beyond dispute by anyone who cares to look at the record. The only question should be whether it is effective. Again, there is ample evidence that chelation therapy is effective.

I do not wish to lay on organized medicine the burden that it is mercenary, nor that it does not care for the best interests of its patients. Nor do I believe that there is an organized attempt to suppress new treatments such as those proposed in this book. In this respect some of my friends say that I am naive, but my experience is that most physicians are much too busy to get involved at that petty level of politics. Physicians are human, though, and some rascals do seem to have made it through the rigors of medical training. Therefore, I am not surprised that an occasional individual will play upon his colleagues' ignorance in enlisting their support to his benefit. Truth, however, will always win in the end and our goal should always be to be on the winning side of truth. *Nevertheless, nutritional and chelation therapy threaten to substantially reduce the cost of health care (translate that "profits") and those who oppose this approach need to give cause why they should be believed. They have a major financial interest in your continuing in poor health and especially in your submitting to their modes of therapy.*

Pharmaceutical firms, especially, have such a financial interest and simply will not spend money investigating a substance that has no potential for their profit. Nor should we expect them to. Congress has recognized this partially through the orphan drug bill. EDTA and DMSO fall into this category since they are orphan drugs and cannot be protected for the benefit of any one company. Since a sizable portion of research dollars comes from these companies, it is not surprising that little research has been done at the major medical centers which survive on those grants. In fact, not only is there no profit in these options, this approach to health would result in a substantial loss of profits to the major pharmaceutical firms. No, do not expect a lot of support from organized medicine, nor from their benefactors.

I am convinced that chelation might prove useful in certain eye diseases, especially macular degeneration and other vascular eye diseases. It is probable that in the best interests of my patients' health, I will someday obtain the additional training necessary to perform this service. Currently, I am studying the options, so to speak, and have not fully committed myself. I am sufficiently convinced that it is only a matter of time before I submit myself again to the services of a chelation physician. And that time will be fairly soon.

It is your right to be well-informed and to demand only the best for yourself. For those who wish to read a well-documented book on chelation therapy, I would like to recommend *Bypassing Bypass*, in the list of recommended reading at the end of this book. This book is written by Dr. Elmer Cranton, a physician with both academic and practical credentials sufficient to merit a fair hearing. Of the various books written on chelation therapy, this is the most current and certainly the most informative. Not a book on how to administer chelation therapy, it is written to both the general public and the practicing physician. Any physician who dismisses the advantages of chelation therapy without giving the evidence a fair hearing does not have your best interests at heart.

8
Free Radical Pathology

Every few generations, an insight comes along so profound that it cuts through the veil clouding our minds and puts into perspective a confusing collection of observations and facts. Mendel's discovery of the basic rules of genetics was one such insight. So was the discovery of bacteria and their role in infection.

Free radical pathology, first put forth by Dr. Denham Harman three decades ago, is such a discovery which promises to tie together a lot of loose ends in degenerative diseases: everything from arthritis and atherosclerosis to diabetes, cancer, and aging.

Free radicals, as used here, is not a term describing members of the Weather Underground who have not been apprehended. A free radical, in its simplest term, is an atom or molecule which has an unpaired electron in its outer shell and is therefore highly reactive. A free radical is an accident looking for a place to happen, so to speak. Free radicals are both essential for life processes and highly destructive to life. Controlled within the mitochondria (organelles within each cell), free radicals release energy for useful work. Free radicals are also a necessary result of detoxifying many chemicals, including drugs, petrochemicals (smog, for example), artificial flavors and colorings, and rancid fats. In fact, your leucocytes (white cells) use free radicals to kill invading bacteria. Outside this controlled environment, free radicals destroy cellular membranes, genetic material, enzymes, and life itself. We are not unaccustomed to such a concept, for the fire contained within a furnace warms the home and soul, but, uncontrolled, the same fire can turn that home into a smoldering pile of ashes. Virtually everything useful is potentially dangerous, even lethal. That is the nature of life. Controlling these forces is what life is all about, at both the molecular and the cellular level as well as at the level of society and the individual.

Since most of the free radicals to which we are exposed are transported via blood, it is only natural that the walls of blood vessels suffer most from their attack. An atheroma, the beginning stage of degenerative blood vessel disease, is essentially a benign tumor growing in the wall of a blood vessel. As it enlarges, it outgrows its blood supply (it must get its nutrients directly from the blood), and necroses (dies) within. This dead tissue within the atheroma accumulates calcium deposits, which further hardens the walls of the blood vessel. The atheroma causes damage by restricting blood flow (which produces anoxia, which produces more free radicals), and by becoming a nidus for the formation of a thrombosis (blood clot) which we have already seen to be activated by free radicals. Once free radical activity is controlled, natural healing processes will diminish the size of any atheroma present.

Malignancy is caused when free radicals react with cellular DNA and alter the genetic material of a cell. If the damage is located at a critical place, the cell multiplies out of control, possibly producing death.

If the free radical damage is to a less critical part of DNA, or to RNA, abnormal enzymes or proteins are produced and cell function is compromised. If the attack is on a cell membrane, the membrane ceases to function and becomes leaky, allowing essential ions to leak out of the cell, or ions which should remain outside the cell to leak in. Loss of cellular chromium in this manner is one cause of adult onset diabetes. The ensuing loss of cellular potassium and magnesium and the influx of sodium and calcium are a major cause of hypertension. (Essential fatty acids which have been altered by food processors also result in leaky cell membranes. Evening primrose oil and borage seed oil are two sources of unaltered essential fatty acids.)

Free radical damage to collagen causes the cross-linkage of collagen molecules and the loss of elasticity. Wrinkled skin, stiff joints, and hypertension are natural results. Silicon in the diet seems to protect collagen against cross-linkage.

In the mitochondria, free radicals are neutralized by an enzyme named superoxide dismutase (SOD). This enzyme contains manganese, which is frequently deficient in the American diet. Outside the mitochondria, another form of SOD is used which contains both zinc and copper. Another scavenging enzyme, glutathione peroxidase, requires four atoms of selenium. Both selenium and zinc are common deficiencies. Free radicals are also produced within the body through reactions in which iron or copper acts as a catalyst. Since both copper and iron are parts of different enzymes which function to scavenge free radicals, they are essential to life. But in excess, both produce free radicals. This property of iron and copper to be both friend and foe makes it urgent that they should never be heavily supplemented without first demonstrating a deficiency by laboratory test.

In addition to the enzymes mentioned above, certain vitamins and elements function as free radical scavengers. Vitamin E's only function may be to intercept free radicals and reduce them to a non-toxic form. In the process, vitamin E is oxidized to tocoperol quinone. Oxidized vitamin E is recycled to tocoperol by vitamin C, which, in turn, is oxidized to dehydroascorbate. Dehydroascorbate is recycled to vitamin C by the enzyme glutathione peroxidase (which requires selenium). Glutathione peroxidase is restored to its active form by oxidizing reduced glutathione, which, in turn, is reduced again by a riboflavin-dependent enzyme, glutathione reductase. This enzyme is reactivated by NADH, a niacin-containing enzyme. The result is oxidized NAD, which enters normal metabolic pathways and produces useful energy or work. NAD itself is synthesized through the action of magnesium, niacin, coenzyme Q-10, and (indirectly) n,n dimethylglycine.

It is important to note that the detoxification of a free radical requires several elements and vitamins, all present and working together. Obviously, if the diet is deficient in one element or enzyme in this complex chain of reactions, supplementing with one of the other elements will produce minimal benefits. It is for this reason that attempts to determine the benefit of isolated nutrients have frequently produced equivocal results. It is as irrational as trying to determine the effect of food while simultaneously depriving the subject of oxygen. The ensuing death may have very little to do with a lack of calories.

Dietary items which are effective free radical scavengers include beta-carotene, vitamin E, vitamin C, selenium (which is effective as an element and in its associated enzyme), cysteine (which is used in the synthesis of glutathione), riboflavin, and niacin. One of the most dangerous free radical forms is singlet oxygen (not paired as the usual oxygen molecule), for which we have no internal defense systems. Singlet oxygen is the result of overloaded internal defense systems (SOD), or exposure to pollutants such as tobacco smoke. The most effective and perhaps only substance for neutralizing the oxygen free radical is beta-carotene, which effectively explains why dietary beta-carotenes are associated with a markedly reduced cancer risk. It is important to note that although beta-carotene is a precursor of vitamin A, vitamin A does *not* have this protective ability. By far the most efficient way to get beta-carotene into your body is to use a juicer and drink carrot juice daily.

Radiation, a major fear among many today, injures and kills through the production of free radicals. The free radicals produced by radiation *are not different* from those produced by rancid foods, pollution, or normal metabolism. In fact, free radicals in our diet and those we internally produce present a much greater risk than we would have encountered by living inside the Three Mile Island nuclear plant at the time of the radiation leak. Free radical pathology is so rampant that aging and degenerative diseases could be considered the end result of an internal nuclear meltdown.

How do free radicals produce such diverse pathologies? In the case of cancer, free radicals reacting with DNA produce an abnormal replication of genetic material, which may result in a malignant transformation. In reacting with lubricants within the joints, or with collagen within tendons and ligaments, there is a reduction in lubrication with the joint or in elasticity of the connecting tissues. The results include joint pains and arthritis. The combination of all these activities of free radicals results in what is commonly called the aging process. If the tissues in the walls of blood vessels are involved, then atherosclerosis is the unavoidable result.

In one situation, peroxidized fats (fatty free radicals) are proven to inhibit an enzyme (prostacyclin) which prevents blood from clotting within a blood vessel. Peroxidized fats, which become concentrated in diseased arterial walls (made that way by free radical damage), increase the probability that a blood clot will form at the diseased site. In the process of clot formation, blood cells rupture and release both iron and copper, which act as catalysts to further peroxidation of fats, which goes through the cycle and causes the clot to extend. This explains why a meal rich in peroxidized fats can trigger a myocardial infarction (heart attack), and why heavy supplementation with vitamin E (which helps prevent the formation of peroxidized fats) will reduce the risk of such attacks (myocardial infarctions, strokes, and venous thrombosis).

There is a simple test to determine the amount of

damage you have sustained from free radicals. Extend your hand, without tightening the skin. Grasp the skin on the back of your hand with your other hand and lift the fold upwards. Release the fold of skin and notice how fast it snaps back into position. In a young person, or anyone with minimal free radical damage, the skin will snap back immediately. When there is considerable damage due to cross linkage of collagen (a connective tissue found throughout the body), the skin fold will slowly slip back into place, sometimes taking several seconds. Try this test on yourself, on a young person's skin, and on an elderly person. The degeneration demonstrated by this test is occurring throughout the body and is reversible by proper nutrition and perhaps, additionally, chelation therapy.

Several years ago, it was noted that persons who have a crease in the skin of the ear lobe are more prone to heart disease. This crease is the result of free radical cross-linkage of collagen molecules.

A third test for free radical damage must be ordered by your physician. Cholesterol is one of the body's defenses against free radicals, and is produced internally in response to free radical levels. Reduced (beneficial) cholesterol is bound to a high density lipoprotein molecule (HDL). When it reacts with a free radical, the peroxidized cholesterol molecule becomes toxic and is bound to a low density lipoprotein molecule (LDL). This toxic cholesterol is removed by the liver and excreted in bile. Vitamin C is essential for its elimination. Dietary fiber is essential to prevent the excreted toxic cholesterol from being resorbed. By testing for total cholesterol and for LDL and HDL cholesterol, the physician can determine your free radical status. Ideally, the LDL should be low, and the majority of your cholesterol should be the reduced type which is bound to HDL. Any level of total cholesterol greater than 150 probably indicates free radical activity, but only levels above 200 are statistically associated with an increased risk of heart disease.

Where are all these free radicals coming from? Certainly, it is not a Communist plot to destroy us all. It is perhaps more a matter of internal subversion and fifth-column activities. As discussed earlier, free radicals are a part of normal metabolism and are controlled within the mitochondria if proper nutrients are available. Without these free radicals we would die, so we will not concern ourselves about them as a separate source.

The major sources of free radicals include natural and man-made radiation (x-rays, gamma rays, and the like), peroxidized dietary fats (*all* unsaturated and rancid fats), ozone, internal oxidation of fats, alcohol (which is metabolized to acetaldehyde, which generates free radicals), aromatic hydrocarbons within tobacco smoke, chlorinated water, and cadmium within drinking water and tobacco smoke. Already mentioned are dietary excesses of iron and copper, which, like cadmium, are free radical catalysts. Anoxia (too little oxygen) produces free radicals. Anoxia, of course, can occur with injury or reduced cardiac/lung function and always occurs when we get insufficient exercise. Hyperbaric oxygen suppresses the free radical process, both directly and by reducing anoxia. Also, hyperbaric oxygen increases the activity of superoxide dismutase (SOD), which in turn helps control free radical activity. In addition, all free radicals catalyze the production of additional free radicals and can increase their concentration a million-fold in seconds. Incidentally, peroxidized cholesterol is an extremely toxic free radical and is bound preferentially to low density lipoproteins (LDL). Reduced cholesterol is a potent scavenger of free radicals (at which time it becomes peroxidized) and is preferentially bound to high density lipoproteins (HDL). An egg yolk in which the yolk membrane is intact is an excellent source of beneficial reduced cholesterol. If the yolk is broken in the cooking process, the cholesterol is oxidized and becomes very toxic. Thus an egg boiled, poached, or sunny-side up is wholesome, whereas it is toxic when scrambled or used in an omelet or cooked in cakes or custards.

Of these sources of free radicals, peroxidized fats are by far the most common and dangerous source. Fats become peroxidized (transformed into free radicals) upon exposure to oxygen (in the air), during metabolism, and especially upon exposure to air while being heated. Fat stored within the body also oxidizes into toxic lipid peroxides, so fat is dangerous when it is eaten and when it is stored as excess weight. Metal ions, especially iron and copper, speed the process. Not only does this combination of factors peroxidize fats, but it also produces an isomerization of the fat molecule which then gets incorporated into cell membranes, producing a defective membrane. But that is another problem, not directly related to free radical damage.

Unsaturated fats, those vegetable oils so highly touted and advertised, are most easily oxidized. To manufacture these oils without toxic peroxidation would require cold pressing in an inert atmosphere devoid of oxygen and in the presence of additional vitamin E. It is possible, but not economically feasible. The worst of all worlds is the re-use of cooking oils, especially for frying and especially where the oil is kept hot for hours on end. This is exactly the situation where fried foods are cooked in fast food restaurants. Obviously, you will use unsaturated oils in preparation of foods. Buy them in small glass containers, use them promptly, and never reuse them. Antioxidants such as BHT could be added to oils to reduce this toxic reaction.

Saturated fats, those found in animal fats and butter, are less easily peroxidized, but will oxidize if the temperatures are high enough. The flavor of grilled meat is due to saturated fats which become peroxidized upon contact with hot charcoal. Nevertheless, saturated fats are safer than unsaturated fats, especially if used in moderation. Butter, a natural saturated fat, is much safer than margarine, which not only contains high levels of peroxidized fats, but also contains those modified fat molecules which produce leaky cellular membranes. So much for good intentions.

Vitamin C appears to be the major defense against free radical damage within the brain, eye, and central nervous system. It is so important, in fact, that there is a natural pump mechanism which increases the concentration of vitamin C in those tissues to many times that in other parts of the body. Anoxia, as caused by stroke, injury, or heart attack, produces a rapid increase of free radicals within the brain to lethal levels. Vitamin C, if present before the injury, will reduce the extent of injury. DMSO, an extremely potent synthetic free radical scavenger, also protects tissue during injury. Hydergine™ (Sandoz) likewise has been proven to delay central nervous system damage during anoxia. Routine administration of vitamin C and Hydergine™ during labor and delivery would probably have very beneficial effects on the health of the child. (Vitamin E does not pass the placental barrier and would not be immediately beneficial, except to the mother.)

Is there any evidence that antioxidant compounds prolong life and reduce aging (and other free radical pathology)? Yes, there is. Mice fed food preserved with antioxidants live longer. More importantly, the effect extends to offspring when the antioxidants are used before mating. Santoquin™, a feed antioxidant made by Monsanto for the poultry industry, displays some interesting effects which may prove the point of argument being made. Specifically, poultry fed Santoquin™ live longer and lay eggs longer than poultry not fed Santoquin™. Santoquin™ is a synthetic vitamin E analog many times more potent than vitamin E as a free radical quencher. Unfortunately, definitive answers will take years to establish.

9
Thyroid Function and Health

By far the most common disease in my experience is thyroid deficiency, which may be present in as many as 40 percent of all adults. A logical question would be why a disease would afflict such a large percentage of the population. The answer is simple. Prior to antibiotics, persons with hypothyroidism died of childhood diseases and therefore had no offspring. With the advent of antibiotics, these children are living to adulthood and raising families. As adults, they are developing the diseases caused by long-term thyroid deficiency, namely atherosclerosis, strokes, heart disease, and cancer. Other probable explanations for chronic hypothyroidism include the toxins in our diet and environment. Many drugs, including aspirin and birth control pills, are toxic to the thyroid gland. Chlorine and fluoride added to municipal water supplies are also toxic to the thyroid gland. Those of us who lived in the fallout pattern of atmospheric nuclear tests in the 1950s were exposed to significant levels of radioactive iodine, which can destroy the thyroid gland; even a tiny dose of radioactive iodine will destroy part of the thyroid gland. (In recent months the U.S. government has been forced to pay for damage due to radioactive iodine near some of the weapons plants. If, however, you expect the government to admit responsibility, you do not understand government.)

The Barnes Basal Temperature Test (BBTT) is simple and accurate. Before going to bed in the evening, shake down an oral thermometer and place it by your bedside where it will be safe from accidental breakage. (Inexpensive electronic digital thermometers are also available and are safer and easier to read.) Immediately upon awakening, take your oral temperature. Record the temperature and repeat several days in a row. *A temperature below 97.5° F indicates probable hypothyroidism.* The test is not accurate if you are ill (with a fever) or during menstruation. *A temperature above 98.2° indicates possible hyperthyroidism* (or fever from an infection). If the test is positive, these other tests may be done by your physician to confirm the diagnosis: thyroid function tests (T3, T4, TSH) and tests for cholesterol levels. However, these tests are chemical tests and are more subject to error than is the BBTT, which has been proven in studies involving several thousand patients. Of the blood tests, the TSH is the most reliable. The diagnosis is confirmed when body temperature normalizes and/or symptoms cease upon treatment.

Symptoms of Thyroid Deficiency:

(A deficiency of the nutrient in parentheses may cause the same symptom.)

- lack of energy (Mg)
- frequent headaches (Mg)
- muscle cramps (Mg)
- dry skin, hair, and eyes (vit A)
- constipation (Mg)
- numbness and loss of nerve function
- loss of memory (Mg)
- all cardio-vascular diseases
- depression (Mg)
- mitral valve prolapse (Mg, Q-10)
- menstrual problems
- cold hands or feet or general cold intolerance
- frequent infections, especially upper respiratory, sinusitis, and of the eyes (all mucous membranes) (vit A)

- loss of color vision (vit A)
- hypoglycemia (chromium)
- slow or weak pulse
- low tension glaucoma
- macular degeneration
- elevated cholesterol
- hypo- or hypertension
- diabetic retinopathy

Persons with two or more of these symptoms, especially those with a low BBTT, deserve a clinical trial of thyroid hormone.

Three eye diseases definitely are associated with hypothyroidism: macular degeneration, diabetic retinopathy, and low pressure glaucoma. In my experience, virtually everyone with any of these diseases is hypothyroid. *Prevention and reversal are possible with a combination of nutritional supplements and thyroid hormone.* In my practice, laser therapy is rarely needed, although laser surgery remains a suitable option for most patients.

The recommended initial treatment is L-Thyroxine, 25 to 50 micrograms each morning. Repeat the BBTT in two weeks and increase the dosage by one tablet until you achieve a normal BBTT. Do not, however, go above 150 mcg of L-Thyroxine daily; only rarely is a higher dose needed. Continue at that level and monitor your BBTT every few weeks until you are certain you are stable. Also have your pulse and blood pressure checked regularly until your maintenance dose is reached. An excessive amount of thyroid hormone will cause your pulse to race and your blood pressure to elevate. Generally, if your resting pulse rate is greater than 85, then you should take thyroid only very cautiously and then only with the close supervision of your physician. Occasionally, the temperature may plateau and remain at a lower level for several months before continuing to rise.

About 20 percent of persons who are low thyroid cannot efficiently convert T4 to T3. T4 is the form of thyroid hormone as it is made and stored in the thyroid gland. It is converted to the active T3 form as the body needs it. T3 is about ten times more potent than is T4. If 150 micrograms of L-thyroxine (T4) does not bring your temperature up to normal, you should cut the dose to 100 micrograms and add Cytomel™ (pure T3) to the dose. Then adjust the dose of Cytomel™.

Persons who have had a recent heart attack or who have cardiac arrhythmias should not use thyroid except under the direct supervision of their family physician or cardiologist. Elevated pulse rates and cardiac arrhythmias are frequently due to magnesium deficiency. Magnesium-potassium aspartate is suggested.

Obviously, patients who are hyperthyroid (as indicated by the BBTT or laboratory testing) should not take supplemental thyroid hormone.

However, work by Broda Barnes, M.D., and others have confirmed that thyroid deficiency is a major cause of atherosclerosis and heart disease. As stated by one researcher, the person with heart disease is better off with a small dose of thyroid hormone than with none. The problem is that in severe heart disease the body can barely tolerate the increased metabolism produced by administering thyroid hormone, even though it is needed. For example, moderate exercise is beneficial for the heart patient; but if the patient has allowed his condition to deteriorate to the point of not being able to walk, what do you do next? The same problem occurs in the end stages of diseases caused by insufficient thyroid hormone. As with exercise, it is frequently possible to restore health slowly by using gradually-increasing doses of thyroid hormone. Persons who have cardio-vascular diseases and also have symptoms of thyroid deficiency and a low BBTT need to be on thyroid hormone, but at a lower initial dose. I initiate therapy for these with 12.5-25 mcg of

L-Thyroxine, then adjust upwards cautiously at one- to three-month intervals. Persons with heart disease are almost universally deficient in thyroid hormone, coenzyme Q-10, and magnesium. Use of all three under medical supervision is strongly advised.

Symptoms of thyroid toxicity include a rapid pulse, nervousness and tremors, and excessive sweating. If these develop while the BBTT is still low, then you most probably have deficiencies of copper, magnesium, or coenzyme Q-10. Reduce your dose of thyroid until these are corrected.

Copper and zinc are necessary for the proper utilization of thyroid hormone. A copper or zinc deficiency can result in symptoms of hypothyroidism, even when serum levels of thyroid are entirely normal. So can a deficiency in coenzyme Q-10 or magnesium, and their use should be seriously considered.

Persons who are hypothyroid will have a vitamin A deficiency and should take 20,000 units of vitamin A daily for three months. In addition, they almost certainly will have moderate to severe mineral deficiencies. A hair analysis is indicated.

Clinical signs of vitamin A deficiency include night blindness, dryness of the eyes, frequent eye infections including chalazions and blepharitis, dry itchy skin especially with a course texture, and a loss of color vision and even a loss of visual acuity. The major food sources of vitamin A are liver, eggs, broccoli, dark green leafy vegetables, and yellow fruit and vegetables.

I cannot legally prescribe thyroid hormone through the mail for anyone whom I have not personally examined. Please understand and do not ask me to do so.

It is imperative that both you and your physician read *Solved: The Riddle of Illness*, by Stephen E. Langer, M.D., *Solved: The Riddle of Heart Attacks*, by Broda O. Barnes, M.D., and *Nutrition, Health, and Disease*, all available from Bio-Zoe, Inc. Also available from Bio-Zoe is a

60-minute lecture on thyroid disease, highly recommended for physicians and anyone who might be hypothyroid.

10

Cholesterol: A Mixed Blessing

If you are approaching middle age and are not yet concerned about cholesterol, you have a marvelous ability to ignore a constant bombardment from television ads, radio, your friends, and your physician. You are being advised to stop eating saturated fats (beef, butter, lard) and switch to unsaturated vegetable fats and margarine. You have been advised to stop eating eggs, which contain a lot of cholesterol, and get your nutrition as best you can.

You have been given bad advice.

Cholesterol is a compound manufactured within your body to meet certain needs of the body. Cholesterol is so important that virtually every cell in the body produces it. It is the starting point for producing hormones, vitamin D, and bile. Without cholesterol, you cannot grow, you cannot digest your food, you will not mature, and you will die. Although the average American diet, rich in cholesterol, supplies about 500 milligrams of cholesterol, your body will synthesize an additional 2000 milligrams daily. If you eat more, you will synthesize less. If you eat less, you will synthesize more. Totally eliminating cholesterol from your diet will not materially affect your blood cholesterol levels. Each egg you eat contains about 250 milligrams of the beneficial HDL form of cholesterol and helps your body by eliminating the need for you to synthesize that amount. You could eat as many as six eggs daily without affecting your blood cholesterol levels if they were properly cooked. So, include up to perhaps two eggs in your daily diet. You need the good nutrition eggs provide. Those foods which are good sources of cholesterol are also very nutritious.

Still, a high blood level of LDL cholesterol (the toxic form) is clearly associated with cardio-vascular disease. If diet does not affect the level of cholesterol in the blood, what will?

It turns out that there are basically two types of cholesterol: a reduced wholesome form and a toxic peroxidized form. The reduced (good) form attaches itself to a high-density lipoprotein (HDL). The toxic peroxidized form is associated with a low-density lipoprotein (LDL) and is excreted via bile if there is enough vitamin C in the diet. In its natural form, egg yolk is a rich source of the good reduced form of cholesterol and is both wholesome and beneficial. If the yolk membrane is broken during cooking or used in a batter mixture, however, the cholesterol quickly oxidizes to the toxic form. For this reason, eggs boiled, poached, or cooked sunny-side up are wholesome, but those cooked scrambled, in an omelet, or in pastry are harmful.

About two decades ago, a study was done in which a group of middle-aged men, all with high blood cholesterol levels, were divided into two groups. One group was put on a low-cholesterol diet; the second group was put on a high-cholesterol diet. Each group was then further divided into two groups each. One group was allowed to continue as before, and the second group was put on an ever-increasing exercise regimen which led to their jogging about a mile daily by the end of the study. The cholesterol levels of those who did not enter into an exercise program remained high; diet had no significant effect on cholesterol levels. Of those who were exercising vigorously, cholesterol levels dropped significantly; again, diet had no real effect. The conclusion is obvious: dietary cholesterol (if in its beneficial reduced form), within reason, will not affect blood cholesterol levels. Even moderate exercise will. Even more significantly, exercise increases the high-density lipid levels while decreasing the low-density lipid levels. This shift is very good.

High blood cholesterol levels could be due to any one of three factors: too much produced, too much ingested, or too little removed from the body. The experiment with exercise clearly shows us that the amount we ingest is of no consequence; the problem lies with over-production or with poor elimination. Both have proven to be important factors.

Elevated cholesterol levels may also indicate hypothyroidism, highly likely since perhaps 40 percent of our population is hypothyroid. I urge you to read Dr. Langer's book (see reading list) for a thorough discussion of this largely ignored disease.

Cholesterol is a potent antioxidant, scavenging from our bodies free radicals, those highly charged molecules which can produce cellular damage, leading to aging and/or cancer. Cholesterol is one of our natural defense mechanisms against this enemy. But only one defense. It should be noted at this point that fat in the diet is a major source of both free radicals and cholesterol; therefore, calories supplied by fat should be reduced to 25 percent, a significant reduction for most of us. Other defenses include vitamin A, beta-carotene, vitamin B_1, (thiamin), vitamin B_3 (niacin), vitamin B_5 (pantothenic acid), vitamin B-6 (pyridoxine), vitamin C, vitamin E, chromium, manganese, silicon, selenium, vanadium, and zinc. Copper and iron are beneficial, but only if there is not an excess. Of these, the only one we can produce within the body is cholesterol; the rest must be part of our diet. Provide the proper nutrients, and your body will not have to manufacture so much cholesterol to defend itself against a hostile environment.

It turns out that the advice to stop eating eggs and to substitute unsaturated oils for saturated fats such as butter has been a serious mistake. First, in eliminating eggs we eliminate excellent nutrition without reducing the cholesterol levels one iota. In addition, we force the body to use precious resources to produce the extra cholesterol needed.

Second, in substituting unsaturated oils for butter and shortening, we substitute a product that is *much* more susceptible to oxidation than the saturated fats. The oxidation of fats produces the very toxic products we should be trying to avoid: namely, the free radicals. Rancid oils are probably the most common source of carcinogens, other than tobacco products, that we are apt to use daily. *In our effort to reduce cholesterol, we have increased the body's need for it.*

L-Carnitine, a vitamin-like substance found in meat, 250 milligrams twice daily, will reduce blood cholesterol levels within two weeks. L-Carnitine is more effective taken with essential fatty acids or Evening primrose oil. The reader should note that D-Carnitine and DL-Carnitine are both toxic; use only the pure L-Carnitine.

Bioflavinoids, especially quercitin, are very effective in reducing blood cholesterol. They are especially effective along with L-Carnitine and essential fatty acids in reducing blood triglycerides.

Several years ago, I decided to abandon my generally low-cholesterol diet and switch from margarine to butter. I also switched to the antioxidant supplement discussed in this chapter. As a result, my cholesterol dropped from 289 to 189, in spite of a weight gain and general lack of exercise during that period of time. By increasing my exercise levels and decreasing my weight, I will improve that figure even more.

Fiber is another means of controlling cholesterol. Toxic peroxidized cholesterol is excreted into the small intestine along with bile which helps in the absorption of fats and fat soluble vitamins. A high-fiber diet will trap a good bit of that cholesterol in the intestine so that it is removed from the body. And, incidentally, additional vitamin C and choline will make the cholesterol more soluble so that gallstones are less likely to be formed. Cholesterol gallstones can also be dissolved using increased quantities of vitamin C and choline. Choline is essential to mobilize and dissolve plaques of cholesterol from blood vessels. The richest source of choline, and the least expensive, is soy lecithin.

Interestingly, the mechanism of lecithin's effectiveness in removing cholesterol deposits may be purely basic physical chemistry. The melting point of cholesterol is well above body temperature. A mixture of alpha-linoleic acid (from vegetable oil) and cholesterol melts right at normal body temperature. A mixture of lecithin and cholesterol melts at about a degree below normal body temperature. Therefore, lecithin tends to dissolve cholesterol deposits by simply liquefying the cholesterol. This simple physical characteristic of cholesterol may also explain why thyroid hormone (which raises body temperature) is so effective in lowering cholesterol levels. Two lecithin capsules daily should be sufficient except in cases of severe cholesterol deposits. Choline, a component in lecithin, is necessary for the liver to process and get rid of cholesterol.

In summary, if you have a high-cholesterol problem, the problem is not one of too much in the diet. The problem may be one of too many free radicals combined with too little physical activity. It may also be due to hypothyroidism, the best test for which is the basal temperature test. If your resting oral temperature is below 97.5° you are hypothyroid, and treatment is indicated. The cure is fivefold. First, work with your physician and set up a gradually increasing program of daily exercise. This is extremely important; not only does it reduce cholesterol and increase the HDL fraction, but exercise is a potent tranquilizer, and stress is known to elevate cholesterol levels. Second, take choline or lecithin liberally to dis-solve the cholesterol deposits from your arteries and mobilize it so that it may be excreted. The least expensive source of choline is lecithin. Two capsules daily are recommended. Third, increase your vitamin C intake to keep the cholesterol soluble and thereby avoid gallstones during the cleansing period. Vitamin C will also reduce your need to keep the cholesterol levels high. As little as 250 milligrams daily is effective, but if you are serious about a cholesterol problem, take at least a gram daily. (Initially, vitamin C will increase blood cholesterol levels as cholesterol deposits are dissolved.) Fourth, increase your intake of the other anti-oxidant nutrients. And, finally, increase your fiber intake. Natural fiber is an excellent source of silicon and also tends to trap the excreted toxic cholesterol so that it is not resorbed. Not all fiber is effective, however—only those natural fibers which contain minerals and perhaps unknown factors. Niacin, 50 to 1300 milligrams (will cause a strong hot flush), taken several times per day, will drastically drop cholesterol levels. One should begin with low levels and gradually increase to tolerance. Niacin is more effective with vitamins E and C and lecithin. Coenzyme Q-10 and n,n dimethylglycine have also been proven to reduce cholesterol levels. Both are natural food products and are totally non-toxic.

Many of these needs can be met by switching your diet away from animal proteins toward a vegetarian diet. I do not advocate a complete vegetarian diet, although that can be very healthy when done properly. What I am suggesting is to make vegetables the main part of your meal, rather than follow the usual American practice of making meat the main course, with vegetables merely an afterthought. The pure vegetarian diet is usually deficient in vitamin B_{12} and in some amino acids. The simplest solution is to eat some animal protein daily. Remember that vitamin B_{12} must come from meat or from a supplement.

It should be obvious that cholesterol is extremely important in preventing cancer and other degenerative diseases and that reducing cholesterol levels without eliminating free radicals will result in damage to the body. Indeed, *every* cholesterol-lowering drug will result in increased risk of cataracts, cancer, liver necrosis, and premature death. A 20-percent increase in mortality risk is the price you'll pay if you go the pharmaceutical route. Nutritional treatment is cheaper, safer, and more effective.

Cholesterol is a blessing involved in the vital functions of every cell. It becomes a curse when environmental pollution, poor diet, and lax health habits force the body to overproduce cholesterol for its own protection. The solution is not to eliminate cholesterol from the diet, but to eliminate the causes for its excess. Our approach to cholesterol should be a classic example of not throwing the baby out with the bath water. High cholesterol is not a disease; it is the result of major insults to our bodies through a lack of physical activity and proper diet. The holistic approach I have described will work and is cheaper and safer than any drug on the market. I challenge you to put this approach to good use in your life.

11

Magnesium

Several published studies have shown that about 88 percent of the American population are magnesium-deficient. Magnesium is one of the most important minerals for human health and is closely allied with thyroid hormone; thyroid deficiency seems to inhibit magnesium adsorption, and magnesium deficiency seems to intensify the symptoms of thyroid deficiency and toxicity. Magnesium is essential for converting food into energy, for burning fat, for memory, and for preventing muscle cramps. Mild magnesium deficiency results in a lack of energy, muscle cramps, tremors, constipation, loss of memory, and depression. Magnesium deficiency may cause migraine headaches. Magnesium deficiency has been proven to increase the risk of a heart attack or stroke by 100 percent, and taking magnesium at the time a heart attack or stroke occurs makes recovery 83 percent more likely. Looking at it another way, if you are taking 300 milligrams of magnesium per day, you are 50 percent less likely to have a heart attack; if you do have a heart attack, you are 83 percent more likely to walk out of the hospital alive. That means *a person taking magnesium is 91 percent more likely to be alive a year from now than he would be otherwise.*

Magnesium deficiency is a known, proven cause of kidney stones. Persons taking 300 milligrams of magnesium plus 10 milligrams of vitamin B6 have been proven in two separate studies (one at Harvard, one at the University of Stockholm) to have 87 percent fewer incidences of kidney stones. In the United States generally, one person in ten will suffer from kidney stones; in the southeastern United States, with its low soil magnesium levels and high-fat diets, the risk is one in five. Since surgery is necessary for many of these sufferers, the cost runs into the millions annually.

Most cases of heart attack and strokes occur because of magnesium deficiency because magnesium deficiency predisposes the arteries to severe spasm. If the spasm lasts three to five minutes, blood clots might occur. The blood clot will convert a minor inconvenience into a stroke or heart attack. Whereas magnesium will prevent the spasm from occurring, vitamin E will prevent the blood from clotting once spasm does occur. Therefore, magnesium and vitamin E taken in adequate amounts (400-1200 I.U. per day) will prevent heart attack and strokes in the vast majority of cases.

Magnesium, vitamin E, and vitamin B6 work together. A deficiency in magnesium will make you more sensitive to toxic side effects of vitamin E and vitamin B6. For example, it is well-known that vitamin E may aggravate hypertension in some patients. However, if you give these patients magnesium also, the vitamin E does not elevate blood pressures. Coenzyme Q-10 and dimethylglycine both also work in conjunction with magnesium.

A rather interesting side effect from intravenous magnesium therapy serendipitously appeared recently in my practice. A patient of mine with severe magnesium deficiency and glaucoma (often itself due to magnesium deficiency) noted after receiving four grams of magnesium intravenously that the tremor from his Parkinson's disease had stopped. The tremor recurred within a week, but again regressed upon magnesium therapy.

There are no reliable blood or serum tests for magnesium deficiency. Magnesium is stored in the cells, and therefore magnesium levels cannot be determined by testing blood. There are several tests being devised for magnesium, the most accurate of which appears to be the hair analysis or the buccal smear. More recently, standards have been established for erythrocyte (red blood cell) and leucocyte (white blood cell) magnesium levels. These tests should prove useful and accurate. More recently, I have discovered that the size of arteries in the eye compared to the size of accompanying veins gives a reliable indication of the *functional* level of magnesium. Generally speaking, if the A:V ratio is 1:1, then the magnesium level in the body is functionally normal. Any reduction of the A:V ratio below 1:1 indicates a magnesium deficiency. If the A:V ratio drops to 1:2, then magnesium deficiency is severe, and the risk of a heart attack or stroke greatly increases. If there are focal spasms—that is, areas in which the arteries are severely constricted—then the risk of a heart attack or stroke due to magnesium deficiency is very great and the need for magnesium therapy either orally or intravenously is urgent. Do not proceed with an exercise program until this is corrected.

For those physicians who may read this book and want to use the A:V ratio as the arteries and veins appear in the eye to determine magnesium deficiency, be aware that beta blockers and calcium channel blockers all also dilate the arteries. This has to be taken into consideration when one estimates the degree of magnesium deficiency. The person taking a drug which dilates the arteries will have a lower magnesium level than is indicated by the appearance of the arteries simply because the size of the artery is being determined more by the effect of the drug than it is by the effect of the magnesium. Magnesium itself is a very powerful calcium channel blocker, and, if your magnesium levels are adequate, it is highly unlikely that you will have either high blood pressure or an irregular heartbeat.

The A:V ratio is altered by drugs which lower blood pressure by causing vasodilation. Very specifically, beta-blockers (Tenormin™, Inderal™, etc.), calcium channel blockers, and, indirectly, tranquilizers. For persons on these drugs, the physician needs to more readily recommend magnesium therapy. On the other hand, vasoconstrictor drugs, such as caffeine and ephedrine, alter the A:V ratio by constricting the arteries. These drug effects must be appreciated to determine the need for magnesium.

Two major sources of magnesium are hard water and dark green and leafy vegetables, chlorophyll itself being almost identical to hemoglobin with magnesium rather than iron. That may explain the benefit of chlorophyll in the diet. When chlorophyll is absorbed into the blood, it drops its magnesium ion and picks up any free iron. Free iron is a major source of free radical activity, so chlorophyll indirectly lowers our free radical burden.

Dietary fat binds with magnesium and prevents its absorption; therefore, a diet high in fat reduces magnesium absorption. Magnesium oxide is poorly absorbed. The best forms of magnesium for oral supplementation are magnesium-potassium aspartate and magnesium orotate. Calcium supplements, especially if taken to excess, will block magnesium absorption. An overdose of oral magnesium will have a laxative effect. If this occurs, simply reduce the dose.

Diuretics and caffeine both cause magnesium loss. This is particularly dangerous since diuretics used to lower blood pressure cause a loss of magnesium, in time causing an increase in blood pressure and an increased risk of heart attack. The short-term effect of diuretic therapy is to reduce blood pressure and to remove excess salt from the body. The long-term effect is to precipitate a heart attack due to magnesium deficiency: persons using a diuretic for several years have a 20 percent higher mortality from heart attack and stroke than those whose blood pressure was not treated with a diuretic. Since magnesium is lost during the excretion of acid, acid-producing foods such as meat result in magnesium loss. Also, acid-producing foods force the body to balance its acidity by dissolving calcium from bone; therefore, a high-protein diet causes the body to need more calcium, which in turn interferes with magnesium absorption. A vegetarian diet produces less acid and therefore requires less calcium to maintain balance.

Magnesium therapy protocol depends upon the severity of the deficiency. A mild, non-symptomatic deficiency may be treated by taking a supplement supplying 300-600 milligrams of magnesium daily as magnesium aspartate. For a moderate magnesium deficiency, oral treatment will probably be adequate; but if the deficiency is symptomatic, intravenous treatment is indicated, especially if symptoms are not relieved within thirty days of oral magnesium treatment. For magnesium deficiency to be classified as severe or critical, you should have one or several symptoms of magnesium deficiency and very severely constricted arteries as seen on eye examination. *Persons falling in this category are at severe risk of myocardial infarction or stroke.* Intravenous therapy is recommended, if at all possible. Until you can find a doctor who does intravenous therapy, by all means take as much magnesium aspartate or orotate orally as you can tolerate, usually 200 to 300 milligrams per dose, two or three times daily.

12
Protocols for Various Diseases of the Eye

This chapter incorporates patient information sheets and treatment protocols used in my office. These sheets are free to my patients and will be mailed for a $2.00 fee to cover postage and handling to anyone requesting them.

My medical specialty is ophthalmology, and therefore the information which follows deals primarily with diseases of the eye. As I have discovered and as we have seen in preceding chapters, optimal health is possible and can be obtained by treating maladies of all parts of the body in ways similar to these treatments of eye disorders. I urge my readers to pursue their own education about—and love for—their bodies and seek medical experts who incorporate these principles in their striving to help you obtain optimal health.

Please note that the recommended supplements are not all used with any single patient. In practice, the treatment is highly individualized, and this information is printed largely for my convenience in writing out a treatment program for a given individual. In many cases it is necessary to also use conventional medical therapy, and in most cases necessary to use conventional medical therapy initially.

Even though I have used these approaches in my clinical practice for over ten years and continue to use them because they work, I cannot *claim* they work because they have not been tested by the double-blind method required by the FDA. However, I use these methods because they have made it possible to avoid surgery in a high percentage of patients who otherwise would have needed surgery (which I am trained to do), and because there appears to be less toxicity.

My thesis is that the human body is wonderfully created, fully capable of healing itself given the proper building blocks of vitamins, minerals, and enzymes. My therapeutic approach is designed to give the body a chance to do just that. If a patient is starving you don't give him drugs; you give him food. Degenerative diseases are largely due to deficiencies in vitamins, minerals, and enzymes. Supplements are merely concentrated foods, given to reverse the effects of selective starvation.

As with all substances, there is some risk of allergic reaction. If you use this information in an effort to treat any disease, you do so at your own risk. No one can predict a rare reaction in any individual.

Cataract Information Sheet

• **Early cataracts** (correctable to 20/50 or better vision).
   • Nutri-Plex™, 2 tablets with meals twice daily for 6-12 months.
   In a one-year clinical trial, Nutri-Plex™ alone was sufficient to reverse or stop the progression of early cataracts, with nearly 100-percent effectiveness.

• **Posterior sub-capsular cataract.**
   This type of cataract greatly interferes with vision, especially with bright lights. It appears to be the result of diabetes, long-term steroid use, possible thyroid deficiency, and/or chromium deficiency.
   • Nutri-Plex™, 2 tablets with meals twice daily for 12 months.
   • GTF chromium (1000 mcg), 1 to 3 tablets per meal for one bottle (100).

• **Nuclear Sclerosis.**
   This type of cataract is associated with aging, and nutritional therapy seems to be effective in slowing its progression. Zinc and selenium, plus Vitamins E, C, and beta-carotenes have been proven to be effective in preventing this type of cataract. (*Arch Ophth* 106:337-340).
   • Nutri-Plex™, 2 tablets with meals twice daily.
   • L-Glutathione, 50 mg, 4 per day for 6-12 months.
   • Selenium, 200 mcg, 3 per day for 12 months.
   • Non-Esterified Vitamin E, 400 I.U. capsules, 1-3 per day.
   • Buffered Vitamin C, 1000 mg per day with meals.

• **Brunescent cataracts.**
   The dark brown color of the brunescent cataract is due to melanin, the same pigment that produces skin color.

Melanin indicates that the lens of the eye is absorbing a large amount of energy and is thought to be associated with exposure to infrared light, ultra-violet light, intense sunlight, or chemicals and substances which produce free radicals. See *Nutrition, Health, and Disease* for complete discussion.

- Nutri-Plex™, 2 tablets with meals twice daily.
- L-Glutathione, 50 mg, 4 per day for 6-12 months.
- Selenium, 200 mcg, 3 per day for 12 months.
- Non-Esterified Vitamin E, 400 I.U. capsules, 1-3 per day.
- Buffered Vitamin C, 1000 mg per day with meals.

• Opalescent cataracts.

A generalized cloudiness of the eyes is highly indicative of metabolic problems, especially diabetes or mineral deficiencies. It can also be due to an excess of milk in persons who are not tolerant of milk products. This type of cataract can be almost completely reversed if treatment is begun soon enough.

- Nutri-Plex™, 2 tablets with meals twice daily for 6-12 months.

• Cortical spoking and water clefts.

These cataracts also indicate nutritional deficiencies and generally stop progressing with nutritional therapy. Reversal of the water clefts is frequent. Reversal of cortical spoking is unlikely.

- Nutri-Plex™, 2 tablets with meals twice daily for 6-12 months.

• Sutural cataracts.

It is along the suture lines that new cells develop. Therefore deficiencies in vitamins and minerals essential for cell division result in cloudiness along the sutural lines. In my experience, these are almost always reversed with a good vitamin/mineral supplement.

• Nutri-Plex™, 2 tablets with meals twice daily.

• **Corneal guttata.**
Corneal guttata indicates disease of the corneal endothelium, and its presence greatly increases the risk of cataract surgery. Cataract surgery is still possible, but carries with it an increased risk. Since January 1989, I have proven that coenzyme Q-10, 90 milligrams per day, improves the function of diseased endothelium, even to the point of reversing corneal edema.
• Coenzyme Q-10, 50 mg, 3 per day for 3 months, then 2 per day.
• Nutri-Plex™, 2 tablets with meals twice daily to help prevent cataracts, since surgery should be avoided.

In a study delivered before the North Carolina Society of Ophthalmology (May 1988), I demonstrated that nutritional therapy of cataracts results in improvement in vision of 88 percent of patients. Although surgery may still be necessary, those who have undergone a nutritional program seem to heal much faster than those who have not.

Note: Modern techniques of cataract surgery and intraocular lens implants are almost universally successful and are not to be feared. However, many patients have surgical contraindications or simply want to avoid surgery and nutritional therapy is highly advised for these.

Macular Degeneration

Macular degeneration is a disease in which central vision fails due to poor circulation or leakage from the vessels underlying the macula. The macula is the central part of the retina, which is to the eye what film is to a camera. The usual progress of the disease is slow, but it may be very fast. Usually, side vision remains unchanged, but central vision may fade to the point where reading is impossible. Patients with macular degeneration frequently notice distortion of vision, with lines being seen as curved or crooked. Other signs of changing macular status include the loss of the foveal reflex, a positive shift in refraction, an increase in astigmatism, and edema of the retina. These signs require an ophthalmologist's evaluation.

One accepted therapy for macular degeneration is laser photocoagulation of leaking blood vessels in the back of the eye, which is successful in about 15 percent of cases. Those who have this surgery do better than those who do not, if it is of a type that can respond. Only evaluation by a retina specialist can determine whether or not the laser therapy might be effective.

An article in *Archives of Ophthalmology* [Vol. 106 (Feb. 1988), pp. 192-198] proves that oral zinc will improve vision in persons with macular degeneration. The dose they used was 200 milligrams of zinc sulfate daily. In my opinion this is far too much and in the wrong form.

From a purely theoretical point of view, vitamins and minerals which affect the health and integrity of small (microscopic) blood vessels or are necessary for vision might favorably affect the course of this disease. I have actively pursued this course of study for a decade with very good results, reporting my findings to the North Carolina Society of Ophthalmology in 1988.

In my practice, I find that the majority of patients with macular degeneration also have subclinical hypothyroidism. These patients respond very favorably to thyroid supplementation. Most physicians are not familiar with this approach to thyroid function and will be hesitant to prescribe thyroid supplements. However, it does work, and its use is supported within the medical literature.

[For symptoms of thyroid deficiency, see Chapter 9.]

In addition, antioxidant vitamins and minerals favorably affect the disease, improving vision in 88 percent of my patients. Obviously, this treatment will not work when permanent damage has been done to the back of the eye by hemorrhage or scars, although presence of these complications does not preclude use of this approach. With treatment, improvement in early macular degeneration may occur within a few weeks. Advanced cases may take up to a year to show improvement. Treatment must be individualized to each patient; therefore, best results are obtained when patients are examined frequently (at three- to six-month intervals).

Recommended Initial Treatment:

• It is absolutely imperative that you **stop smoking**.

• **Discontinue the use of margarine** and substitute butter.

• **Drink only quality water**—distilled, spring or well, bottled, or purified through a Bone Charcoal filter.

• **Nutri-Plex™**, 2 capsules twice a day with meals.

• **Coenzyme Q-10** (50 mg), two per day.

• **n,n Dimethylglycine (DMG)** (125 mg), 2 per day sublingually.

• **Selenium chelate** (200 mcg), 3 per day for 12 months.

• **Bioflavinoids,** or Quercitin (1000 milligrams), 2 per day.

• **Pycnogenol** (25 mg), 1-2 capsules, 2 times a day on an empty stomach.

• **Earth Food**™ (1 ounce per gallon of distilled water), 4 ounces of this mixture 3-4 times per day.

Recommended Adjunctive Treatment if edema is present:

• **Bioflavinoids,** or Quercitin (1000 milligrams), 2 capsules per day.

Occasionally the following additional nutrients prove useful:

• **Non-esterified natural vitamin E** (400 IU), 3 per day.

• **L-Glutathione** (50 mg), 4 per day until selenium levels are normal.

• **Cod liver oil** (capsule supplying 10,000 IU of vitamin A and 400 IU of vitamin D), 1 daily for 2 months.

• **B6** (500 mg) **with magnesium** (25 mg), 3 capsules per day.

• **Borage seed oil**, 1 capsule daily with a meal.

• **Lecithin** capsules, 2 per day.

• **Zinc picolinate** (20 mg), 2 per day for 2 bottles.

• **Chromacin™ GTF Chromium** (200 mcg), 1-3 per day for 4 months.

• **Magnesium-potassium aspartate**, 2-6 per day at meals or at bedtime.

• **Shark cartilage** capsules, 8 per day for 2 months then 6 per day. Can be effective in reducing neovascularization.

Nutrition in Cataracts and Macular Degeneration

In March 1990, Storz, through its pharmaceutical subsidiary Laderle, sent to every ophthalmologist nationwide reviews of 18 scientific studies proving that nutrition reduces the incidence of cataracts and improves vision in patients with macular degeneration.

I have been successfully using nutrition in treatment of macular degeneration and cataracts since 1979. My results, delivered in a paper before the North Carolina Society of Ophthalmology in 1988, demonstrate that *over 88 percent of patients with macular degeneration or cataracts experienced improved vision with nutritional supplementation.* In practice, each patient must be treated individually, since the deficiencies vary from person to person. I use a hair analysis to determine the relative concentration of various trace elements in the hair, since these trace elements have been proven to be essential in nutrition of the eye and because the hair analysis is both less expensive and a more accurate means of assessing tissue levels of these specific minerals than are blood studies. In macular degeneration, subclinical hypothyroidism is common (almost 90 percent) and thyroid hormone is used for most of these patients. This requires a prescription and cannot be given without the physician actually examining the patient.

The studies cited in the brochure sent out by Laderle include:

1. Newson, D.A. "Oral Zinc in Macular Degeneration." *Arch Ophthalmol* 106 (1988): 192-198.

2. Karcioglu, Z.A. "Zinc in the Eye." *Surv Ophthalmol* 27 (1982): 114-122.

3. Leopald, I.H. "Zinc Deficiency and Visual Impairment?" *Am J Ophthalmol* 85 (1978): 871-875.

4. Russell, R.M. "Zinc and the Special Senses." *Ann Intern Med.* 99 (1983): 227-239.

5. Solomons, N.W. "The Interaction of Vitamin A and Zinc: Implications for Human Nutrition." *Am J Clin Nutr* 33 (1980): 2031-2040.

6. Yolton, D.P. "Nutritional Effects of Zinc on Ocular and Systemic Physiology." *J Am Optometr Assn* 52 (1981): 409-414.

7. Bhat, K.S. "Plasma Calcium and Trace Metals in Human Subjects with Mature Cataract." *Nutrition Reports International* 37 (1988): 157-163.

8. Dwivedi, R.S. "Role of Lipid Peroxidation and Trace Metal in Cataractogenesis." *Ind J Ophthalmol* 34 (1986): 45-51.

9. Fischer, P.W.F. "Effect of Zinc Supplementation on Copper Status in Adult Man." *Am J Clin Nutr* 40 (1984): 743-746.

10. Leure-Dupree, A.E. "Changes in Retinal Morphology and Vitamin A Metabolism as a Consequence of Decreased Zinc Availability." *Retina* 2 (1982): 294-302.

11. Hoyt, C.S., III. "Vitamin Metabolism and Therapy in Ophthalmology." *Surv Ophthalmol* 24 (1979): 177-190.

12. Young, R.W. "Solar Radiation and Age-Related Macular Degeneration." *Surv Ophthalmol* 32 (1988): 252-269.

13. Tso, Mom. "Pathogenetic Factors of Aging Macular Degeneration." *Ophthalmology* 92 (1985): 628-635.

14. Jacques, P.F. "Antioxidant Status in Persons with and Without Senile Cataract." *Arch Ophthalmol* 106 (1988): 337-340.

15. Bunce, G.E. "Cataract—What is the Role of Nutrition in Lens Health?" *Nutrition Today*, Nov/Dec 1988: 6-12.

16. Larsen, P.D. "Vitamin E Deficiency Associated with Vision Loss and Bulbar Weakness." *Ann Neurol* 18 (1985): 725-727.

17. Organisciak, D.T. "The Protective Effect of Ascorbate in Retinal Light Damage of Rats." *Invest Ophthalmol Vis Sci* 26 (1985): 1580-1588.

18. Weiter, J.J. "Relationship of Senile Macular Degeneration to Ocular Pigmentation." *Am J Ophthalmol* 99 (1985): 185-187.

The graphs below show my results in a two-year study presented before the North Carolina Society of Ophthalmology. In each graph, the light color represents the visual acuity of eyes before treatment. The dark gray represents the visual acuity of eyes after treatment. The shift toward the 20/20 line represents improvement. The studies cited and the data presented on this sheet prove conclusively that nutrition is a factor in both cataract formation and in macular degeneration. My clinical studies prove without doubt that visual acuity in cataractous and macular degeneration patients can be improved using nutrition.

Graph No. 1 represents pre- and post-treatment vision of cataract patients. Eighty-eight percent improved. Graph No. 2 represents pre- and post-treatment visual acuity in macular degeneration patients. Two eyes became worse, five remained the same, and 53 (88 percent) improved.

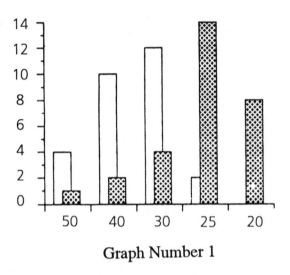

Graph Number 1

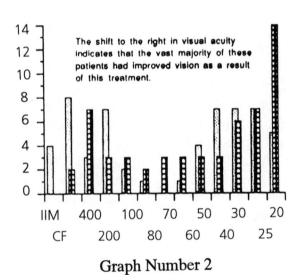

The shift to the right in visual acuity indicates that the vast majority of these patients had improved vision as a result of this treatment.

Graph Number 2

Diabetes Information Sheet

Diabetes Mellitus is a disease in which the patient cannot properly handle carbohydrates, so that the blood levels of glucose rise dangerously. Diabetes follows a distinctly hereditary pattern, although many who have it have no family history of diabetes. Diabetics have an increased risk of atherosclerosis, heart attacks and strokes, kidney disease, cataracts, and blindness. Most of these vascular problems associated with diabetes are actually the result of subclinical hypothyroidism, the treatment for which is discussed in my thyroid information sheet.

It is imperative that individuals with diabetes mellitus be examined by an ophthalmologist (M.D.) at least annually. Blood vessel changes in the back of the eye, if not promptly treated, can lead to blindness.

The diabetic is strongly urged to obtain a copy of my book *Nutrition, Health, and Disease* and study the chapter on diabetes. Additional information is found in my audio tape on diabetes. The steps outlined in that chapter should enable most mild to moderate diabetics to come off insulin and live normal lives without the risk of further complications. *The diabetic should be aware that if he undergoes a program such as being suggested here and in my book, that his insulin or oral antidiabetic medication dosage must be monitored carefully and adjusted accordingly.* Otherwise, there is a distinct risk that he may suffer from insulin shock and other complications.

Body fat requires perhaps five times as much insulin as muscle, and physical exercise tends to reduce the insulin requirement. Therefore, it strongly behooves the diabetic to lose weight and to exercise regularly. By losing weight you will reduce your insulin demand, and by exercising you will use up excess glucose without the need for insulin. The importance of regular exercise and loss of weight cannot be overemphasized. Avoid white sugar, white flour, and white bread. Vegetables and fruit should be eaten unprocessed and raw if possible, and fried foods should be avoided. It is imperative that you stop smoking and discontinue the use of margarine. You may substitute butter.

Specific Recommendations for initial therapy:

•**Hair Analysis.** Aggressively correct deficiencies of zinc, copper, chromium, selenium, magnesium, and manganese.

• **Obtain an electronic glucose meter** such as the Ames Glucometer II so that blood glucose levels can be monitored closely at home.

• **GTF chromium,** __ 200 mcg/ __ 1000 mcg, __ times before meals plus one at bedtime for __ bottles.

•**Nutri-Plex™,** 2 tablets twice daily with meals for 6-12 months.

• **Borage Oil,** one capsule daily.

Adjunctive therapy:

• **Biotin,** 1000 micrograms per day, has been proven to reduce insulin requirements and blood sugar levels in some diabetics.

•**Super C Ascorbs™, or Poten-C™,** __ per day with meals.

• **n,n dimethylglycine (Pure DMG™),** 2 per day, sublingually. This is clinically proven to reduce insulin requirements by as much as 20 percent.

•**Bioflavinoids,** or Quercitin, up to 1000 milligrams per day.

• **Non-esterified natural Vitamin E**, 400 I.U. capsules per day.

• **Eat cold water ocean fish** or trout three times per week to supply necessary fish oils. Cod liver oil, 1 Tbs per day, is equally effective.

Additional therapy for persons with diabetic retinopathy:

• **Borage seed oil**, 1 capsule per day with meal.

• **Shark cartilage**, 8 capsules daily for 2 months then 6 capsules per day.

• **n,n dimethylglycine (DMG)**, 2-4 daily, sublingually or orally.

• **Nutri-Plex™**, 2 tablets twice daily with meals.

• **Garlic** (cloves or capsules) twice daily.

• **Vitamin A & D** (cod liver oil), __ capsules per day for __ bottles.

• **L-Carnitine**, 2 capsules per day plus 1 Borage oil capsule once daily may prove to be very beneficial. This will dramatically lower triglyceride levels and blood fat levels.

• **Sun Chlorella**, 5 tablets per meal for 6 months.

• **Barley Green™**, 1 teaspoon twice daily in water.

Dry Eye Syndrome Information Sheet

Human tears are very complex, not a simple salt water solution layered upon the eye. Human tears actually have three layers: an inner layer of saline which wets the cornea, an outer layer of oil which keeps the tear film intact and prevents evaporation, and a bipolar mucin layer sandwiched between. Oil and water do not mix; therefore, the third layer is necessary to hold the two together. This middle layer consists of molecules, one end of which is soluble in water and the other end of which is soluble in oil.

Dry eye syndrome occurs whenever the cornea tear film dries, exposing the cornea to air. This gives rise to symptoms of blurred vision, scratchiness, and occasionally outright pain. Usually, however, the eyes simply have a feeling of lack of lubrication, and the eyelids seem to stick to the eyes during a blink. In most cases this is due to a lack of the oily film layer. Since vitamin A is an essential component of the oily film, vitamin A deficiency directly results in a tear film defect and the symptoms of dry eyes. Once the eye has dried to the point that the eye feels scratchy, the body reacts with reflex tearing.

Reflex tears, the type we produce when we get something in our eyes, or when we are crying, consist primarily of a salt solution. It is produced in large quantity to wash the offending material out of the eye. A person with dry eye syndrome may have the symptoms of a foreign body in the eye, and will react with reflex tearing. As a result, many persons with dry eye syndrome actually tear a lot.

Traditionally, treatment of dry eye syndrome has been directed toward either replacing the tears with artificial substances or plugging up the drainage holes so that whatever tears are produced do not drain away. Many artificial tear products are on the market, and most seem to be satisfactory, depending on the severity of the situation. The older products such as Liquifilm Tears™ or Liquifilm Forte™ merely add to the eyes a viscus solution that remains there for a long time, since it drains out poorly. Newer products such as Neo-Tears™ or Hypo-Tears™ mimic the three-layered composition of natural tears and are preferred.

Mechanically plugging the drainage holes is accomplished either with a gel or a silicone plug which is used to temporarily plug the punctum in order to determine whether or not this treatment might be beneficial. More drastic, and less likely to be reversed, are surgical procedures which close the drainage opening either by cautery or by laser.

In my own practice, none of the above procedures are used, since none seem necessary. Listed below are measures which generally work, listed in the order of trial, from mildest cases to more severe. Only after these have failed do I resort to lubricating drops.

Suggested Therapy (in order of increasing effectiveness):

• **Discontinue the use of margarine** and use butter instead. Margarine interferes with the synthesis of an important prostaglandin (hormone-like substance) which seems to be necessary for normal tear film development.

• **Nutri-Plex™**, 2 tablets twice daily. This is a comprehensive vitamin-mineral supplement recommended to eliminate the likelihood of major deficiencies.

• If you are not currently not eating liver once a week, then take **A & D capsules**, 1 per day for 1-2 bottles. This is our cod liver oil containing about 10,000 units of vitamin A per capsule. If you wish to take cod liver oil straight, take one tablespoon per day.

- Determine whether or not you are thyroid deficient. Thyroid hormone is essential for conversion of vitamin A to the form that is used in the eye. Thyroid deficiency is a distinctly possible cause of dry eye syndrome. If your body temperature upon awakening is below 97.5°, then it is possible that you are thyroid deficient.

- **Borage seed oil**, 1 capsule per day with meals.

Certain drugs, especially antihistamines and those used to treat allergies and sinusitis, have as a side effect a reduction in tear formation. Obviously, before adding additional drugs you should discontinue the ones that are causing you harm.

If all of the above fail, then seriously consider the use of a lubricating drop. Do not use any drops with a vaso-constrictor or chemical designed to "get the red out." Generally speaking, drops which have the word "tears" in the label are safe for continuous use. Several products which are preservative-free are available, and preferred.

Dry eye symptoms are much worse in the winter due to the drying effect of heated air. This is especially true in homes heated with wood or electric baseboard heating. A good humidifier is essential, and especially recommended are the ultrasonic types. Dressing warmly is preferred to overheating your home. Not only will you save money, but you will find that you will be healthier and have fewer problems with dry eyes.

Glaucoma Information Sheet

Basically there are four types of glaucoma:

Angle closure glaucoma must be treated surgically, usually with a laser.

Pigmentary glaucoma is a variant of open angle glaucoma and responds very poorly to nutritional therapy. Unfortunately, it also responds poorly to all the other various modes of treatment. Usually, however, control is possible and vision is maintained.

Low tension glaucoma is a disease in which nerve damage and visual field loss occur, but eye pressures are normal or even low. It is currently unresponsive to most treatment modalities. It is my experience that low tension glaucoma is actually a disease of sub-clinical hypothyroidism. Many patients whom I have treated thusly have responded with reduced nerve damage and, in many cases, recovery of visual field loss.

The only type of glaucoma for which nutritional therapy might be beneficial is **open angle glaucoma**. It has already been proven that most patients with open angle glaucoma have a deficiency in vitamin A. (*Glaucoma*, December 1983). Certain nutrients are known to reduce abnormal deposits of mucopolysaccharides, which plug the drainage holes in glaucoma patients. Glaucoma patients also have significant deficiencies of the enzyme NAD. This enzyme is related to energy production, and administration of NAD by injection does lower intraocular pressure. However, NAD levels apparently can be boosted by increasing levels of magnesium, coenzyme Q-10, and adenosine triphosphate (ATP). ATP levels can be increased by the use of n,n DMG.

Glaucoma has a definite inheritance pattern. Therefore, if you have glaucoma, it is extremely important that your children, parents, brothers, and sisters be tested for glaucoma by an eye physician.

In my experience, about one out of two cases of open angle glaucoma can be controlled with the following protocol. First, evaluate thyroid function using the Barnes Basal Temperature Test, since persons with low thyroid are unable to utilize vitamin A and deposit mucin in the tissues. If this test proves to be positive, then administration of thyroid is necessary. Second, use a hair analysis to determine the status of micronutrients, especially copper, magnesium, manganese, selenium, and zinc. All of these elements are essential either in a system of detoxification which neutralizes free radicals or in the production of NAD.

Recommended Initial Therapy:

• **Evaluate thyroid function** and treat if indicated.

• **Nutri-Plex™**, 2 tablets twice daily with meals. This supplies basic nutrients and magnesium.

• **n,n dimethylglycine** (DMG™), 1 per day sublingually.

• **Coenzyme Q-10** (50 mg), __ per day.

• **Vitamin A & D** (cod liver oil), 1 per day for 1 bottle.

Recommended Adjunctive Therapy:

• **Biotin** (1000 mcg), 1 per day.

• **Magnesium aspartate chelate** (100 mg), 2-6 per day with meals or at bedtime. Use this if the fundus A:V ratio is less than 1:3.

• **Earth Food**™, 1 oz. per day.

Laser surgery (by a qualified ophthalmologist) is effective for angle closure glaucoma and open angle glaucoma, in selected cases. Other surgical procedures are available and effective. Concurrent surgery for glaucoma and cataract is possible. Fortunately, loss of vision is a rare event with the combination of modern medications, nutritional support, and surgery.

Persons with glaucoma should continue with their medical treatment for at least three months before attempting to taper off and discontinue the treatment. It is extremely important to continue medical management and routine follow-up examinations at three- to six-month intervals under the care of an ophthalmologist even if the nutritional approach completely reverses the glaucoma. The long-term benefits of nutritional therapy for glaucoma is unknown, and caution is advised.

Migraine Information Sheet

Migraine is a peculiar disease that affects the blood vessels. At the beginning of an attack, they squeeze down very tight and remain this way until they are totally exhausted. Then they expand greatly and allow a large volume of blood to rush into the area they supply. During the period of time in which they are constricted, you may have a funny feeling that you are going to get a headache, may feel nausea or actually vomit, and may have visual symptoms such as dancing lights or flashing lines. When the blood vessels dilate, you may have a throbbing headache.

The tendency toward migraine is inherited. There are three parts to the migraine triad: visual symptoms, headaches, and nausea or vomiting. Sometimes patients will have severe stomach cramps. Any one, two, or all three may occur together. Usually the attack will last 15 to 30 minutes but in severe cases may last hours to several days.

For most persons, the headaches can be prevented by a change in lifestyle and diet. You may find that certain foods will trigger an attack. These most commonly are coffee or tea, bananas, seafoods, and hot, spicy foods. Chocolate is an offender for some people. Soy sauce can trigger headaches in an attack called the Chinese Restaurant Syndrome. Other common allergens include beef, wheat, milk, eggs, poultry, potatoes, tomatoes, peppers, and soybeans. If you are troubled by migraine, you should make sure that you get an adequate amount of rest and exercise daily. Avoid stressful situations if at all possible. You are advised to keep a food diary to help identify offending foods.

Mild hypothyroidism is also a recognized cause of migraine headaches. In fact, hypothyroidism is the underlying cause of 95% of frequent headaches and should not be ignored. If your oral temperature is below 97.5° upon awakening, ask for a copy of our Thyroid Information Sheet.

Diet change also includes the addition of bran cereals to the diet. Fortunately, many brands are currently available since the cereal industry has discovered they can make something wholesome. I would like to strongly suggest the frequent use of rolled oats and farina. Shift your diet to include whole fruit. Fill up on vegetables rather than meats and processed foods. Highly refined foods such as white bread and sugar should be eliminated or minimized. Natural yogurt (look for "active yogurt cultures" on label) may be tried. These dietary changes will eliminate headaches for up to 80 percent of persons bothered by migraine.

Certain vitamins and minerals may be effective in preventing migraine attacks. Consider especially magnesium-potassium aspartate, since magnesium is necessary for the relaxation of blood vessels. Manganese may also be effective, but obtain a hair analysis before taking supplemental manganese. B-complex formulas containing at least fifty times the RDA is frequently effective. Of these, niacin seems to be the key vitamin. Vitamin A deficiency seems to be a factor in some. Refer to my Vitamin A Information Sheet.

Gamma linolenic acid is used by the body to produce a hormone-like substance which may prevent migraine headaches. The body can synthesize its own gamma linolenic acid if the diet supplies adequate levels of essential fatty acids, if thyroid levels are functionally adequate, and if the diet supplies adequate amounts of vitamin E and selenium. The best sources of the linoleic acid used in the synthesis process are oils such as safflower oil or corn oil. There are some oils which contain pre-formed gamma linolenic: these include borage seed oil, black currant seed oil, and black walnut oil. Of these, the borage oil is the richest source of gamma linolenic acid. Incidentally, the synthesis of gamma linolenic acid is interfered with by margarine, a major reason why I strongly recommend that persons not eat margarine, but shift rather to butter. If you suffer from migraine headaches, then by all means stop using margarine and hydrogenated fats, and begin consuming an oil rich in gamma linolenic acid, using perhaps one capsule a day of borage seed oil or the equivalent. Once you are confident this has been beneficial, then find your maintenance dose which should be one capsule per day.

If these measures fail, there are several medications that can be effective. The medication used will vary from patient to patient and the pattern that the migraine attack takes. If you continue to suffer from migraine attacks after using these natural approaches, please make an appointment with me and I will prescribe the correct medication. Generally, migraine attacks begin in the early teens and end by age 30. Hormones and birth control pills will trigger migraine attacks and should not be used by any person with migraine. Birth control pills are particularly dangerous for persons with migraine, and such people often have complications with the pills. If you have migraine attacks and are taking birth control pills, you are strongly advised to consult with your family physician for advice on birth control.

Finally, migraine headaches can be caused by a Candida albicans infection in the intestines. Candida infections are most common in persons who have frequently taken antibiotics and in those whose diet contains a lot of sugar and white flour products. *The Yeast Connection*, a book written for Candida sufferers, is highly recommended. In general, if you do have an overgrowth of Candida albicans, the toxic effects are from chemicals produced by the yeast when the yeast is digesting the food you have eaten. Many bizarre symptoms have been attributed to Candida overgrowth. I personally know of patients who had gotten down to the point of being able to eat only five foods and yet had complete relief after the

Candida infestation was killed off. Obviously, they had to avoid processed foods thereafter.

In my experience, the majority of migraine patients can be relieved with a combination of the suggestions made in this information sheet. You will have to essentially become your own physician and become a detective to isolate what is triggering your attacks, and then develop a strategy to prevent them. That is the bad news. The good news is that you probably will be successful.

Subconjunctival Hemorrhage
Information Sheet

A subconjunctival hemorrhage is usually a spontaneous rupture of a tiny blood vessel over the white of the eye, which, due to the confined space of the membranes covering the eye, causes a very large red blot on the eye. Even a tiny drop of blood in the eye looks like a huge amount. Do not be alarmed; even the most massive subconjunctival hemorrhage represents only one or two drops of blood.

In most cases, the redness of the eye will clear completely within 2-6 weeks. If you continue vigorous activities for several days after the initial hemorrhage, the clot will possibly break free, causing additional hemorrhaging. This is not a cause for alarm, but is a cause for caution and cutting back on your activities. A cold compress applied firmly to the eye and held there for five minutes or more may stop the bleeding.

Take 1000-2000 milligrams of vitamin C plus 1000-2000 milligrams of bioflavinoids to make the blood disappear more rapidly. In milder hemorrhages, a combination product such as Poten-C alone will do the job. Take 1-4 tablets per day in divided doses. During the time that the hemorrhage resolves, the color will change from red to greenish-yellow to yellow and finally to white.

The following factors can be a cause of subconjunctival hemorrhages and should be eliminated as causes by proper follow-up examinations. Even with a careful work-up, most cases of subconjunctival hemorrhage remain due to unknown causes.

Causes of subconjunctival hemorrhage:

Trauma or straining. Frequently, subconjunctival hemorrhages occur upon straining as one might in moving furniture or heavy objects, or with constipation.

Infections. Certain bacterial and viral eye infections produce subconjunctival hemorrhages. These should treated by an ophthalmologist (M.D.).

Retinal venous engorgement. This is due to constriction of the outflow passages for blood leaving the eye, resulting in increased venous pressure. This one is potentially serious and should be checked by an ophthalmologist. Treatment is with vitamin E, vitamin C, and other substances which might reduce blood viscosity.

Vitamin C and bioflavinoid deficiency. These vitamins are involved in reducing capillary fragility and their deficiency increases the likelihood of hemorrhages and bruising. If your diet is deficient in these vitamins, supplementation or a change of diet is advised. Generally, at least 500 mg of vitamin C and 250 mg of bioflavinoids are recommended.

Diabetes. Diabetes results in increased capillary fragility and subsequent hemorrhages. If you have not had a check-up for diabetes or if you have a family history of diabetes, you should arrange with your family physician for this to be done.

Hypertension. Hypertension results in increased capillary fragility and subsequent hemorrhages. If you have not had a check-up for hypertension, you should arrange with your family physician for this to be done.

Hypothyroidism. Chronic hypothyroidism results in capillary fragility. If you have a low body temperature (below 97.5° F upon awakening) or are chronically tired, have cold hands and feet or other symptoms of low thyroid, you should obtain a copy of my thyroid information sheet and do what it says. Thyroid deficiency can be treated only by prescription thyroid hormone.

Essential fatty acid deficiency. Essential fatty acids are obtained by eating a diet rich in unsaturated vegetable oils. Margarine and other hydrogenated fats interfere with the utilization of essential fatty acids and may be a cause of subconjunctival hemorrhage. The best way to obtain essential fatty acids is to include in your diet adequate quantities of nuts, seeds, whole grains, and oily fruits such as avocado. The use of margarine should be discontinued. Butter does not supply essential fatty acids, but it at least does not interfere with their use.

Vitamin E and selenium deficiency. A deficiency of either vitamin E or selenium results in malformed and fragile capillaries. In my recent study of over 800 patients, well over 90 percent of patients are deficient in selenium. Most persons would find themselves in better health if they were taking at least 400 units of natural vitamin E and at least 200 micrograms of selenium.

Chromium deficiency. Chromium is essential for the formation of arteries and may also be essential in the formation of healthy capillaries. All diabetics are chromium deficient. Your daily supplementation should include at least 200 mcg of true GTF chromium.

Vitamins and minerals work together. Therefore, you should take a balanced therapeutic formula such as Bio-Zoe's Nutri-Plex™ formula.

Hypoglycemia Information Sheet

Hypoglycemia is a condition in which the blood sugar drops extremely low several hours after a meal rich in sugar or carbohydrates. When the blood sugar is low, you may tremble or feel weak and may also exhibit some bizarre behavior. Diagnosis is generally by a careful history, but it can be done by a six-hour glucose tolerance test. A three- or four-hour glucose tolerance test is not sufficient.

The mechanism is fairly well understood. When you eat a meal high in sugar, your blood sugar will rise fairly rapidly, causing your body to release insulin to keep it from rising too high. If you are deficient in chromium, then insulin will be ineffective, resulting in a higher blood sugar spike than otherwise would occur. After the insulin has begun to take effect, the blood sugar will drop very rapidly, and when it reaches around 60 milligram percent, the liver will start producing sugar from glycogen. The liver can produce sugar only if your thyroid output is adequate. Therefore, when one looks at the overall picture, hypoglycemia can occur if you have a low blood chromium level or a low thyroid level.

Treatment consists primarily of taking GTF chromium supplements, 3-5 200-microgram tablets per meal for 4-5 bottles (100 tablets per bottle) and taking supplemental thyroid hormone, if indicated. In my opinion, the most accurate means of determining whether or not your thyroid is inactive is to take your body temperature by mouth immediately upon awakening in the morning. If it is below 97.5° F, you probably need to be given a prescription for thyroid hormone. Additional information is found on the thyroid information sheet.

[For symptoms of thyroid deficiency, see Chapter 9.]

Therapeutic Options:

One therapeutic option frequently recommended is to switch from eating three large meals a day to many small meals a day, about two hours apart. This works because you do not overload the system with a large amount of carbohydrate at one time; therefore, the blood sugar does not rise high enough to trigger a large insulin release.

An article in *The Journal of the American Medical Association* in 1983 proves that chromium in moderate doses will relieve the symptoms of hypoglycemia.

• **Chromacin™ GTF chromium** (200 mcg), 2-6 tablets per day with meals for 3-5 bottles.

• **Chromacin™ GTF chromium** (1000 mcg), 3-9 tablets per day with meals for 1 bottle.

• **Nutri-Plex™**, 2 tablets twice daily, with meals. There is enough chromium in this formula to correct chromium deficient hypoglycemia.

• Many physicians recommend **many small meals** rather than three larger meals daily. Small meals reduce the amount of insulin released and may avoid hypoglycemia.

Appendix
Emotional and Spiritual
Aspects of Optimal Health

To be truly healthy, a person must be at peace with himself, his God, and his fellow man. It is not possible to love God, for example, and hate yourself, whom God loves. A healthy person will treat others as he would wish to be treated, but not better. It is not a sign of health to continually run oneself down.

The person who desires to be healthy should develop a close and comfortable relationship with God. As this relationship develops, he will come to know that he is accepted by God and therefore should accept himself. After all, if God has accepted you, who are you to argue?

God has said, "You shall be holy, for I am holy." *Holy* means *healthy*. Therefore, we must conclude that the will of God is for us to be healthy. The word *salvation* as used by Christians literally means *healthy*. Therefore, when the New Testament says, "Believe in the Lord Jesus Christ and you shall be saved," it literally means that if you believe in the Lord Jesus Christ you shall be made healthy.

Why then are so many still sick, if this is true? Primarily because most of us have never heard the Gospel to know what it means. Also because we persist in doing things which harm our health even though we know better.

I have written a book, *The Eternal Triangle*, which deals in depth with the spiritual aspects of health. It is a book of considerable depth, forged as it was on the anvil of God's presence and love over a period of more than forty years. If you are satisfied with simple answers, or if you are totally satisfied with your present relationship with God, this book is not for you. However, if you thirst for a deeper relationship with the Father, this book will profoundly affect your life and change forever your relationship with God, your neighbor, and even yourself. In *The Eternal Triangle*, I have attempted to discover and understand the original gospel that turned the Roman Empire upside down and created Western civilization. *That* gospel obviously had power.

Physicians and ministers have known for centuries that attitude affects health. Two stories will illustrate this point. About three years before my father's death, I visited him in September. By that time his health had deteriorated to the point that he could not walk from his bedroom to the bathroom without a walker and assistance. I sat by Dad's bed and told him, "Dad, you and I both know you won't live to see Thanksgiving. In this life there are only two ways to go: each day you are either healthier than the day before, or each day you are one step closer to the grave. It's your choice. If you want to turn this around, then each day walk ten steps more than you did the day before." On Thanksgiving Day, Dad and I walked four miles through the woods and pasture on the farm, Dad using only a cane. Our farm has some fairly rugged terrain, which makes this even more remarkable. Dad had listened.

When my grandfather's first wife died, he had been using a cane for several years. Later, the husband of his childhood sweetheart died, and they decided it wasn't good for both of them to be lonely and set the wedding date. His younger daughter couldn't stand for her Dad to marry again and decided to fix his little red wagon, hiding his cane on his wedding day. Poppa Rainey didn't ask for the cane and never used a cane the rest of his life! Several years later, when his second wife died of cancer, he died in grief within hours of making the funeral arrangements.

They died within hours of each other, having lived their last years in joy.

It has been known for centuries that our attitude toward others affects our own health. How many people suffer from ulcers and hypertension because of their anger at their jobs, fellow workers, or families? The body in many ways reacts to our emotional health. For example, people who feel that they are carrying burdens frequently complain of back aches. A friend of mine who had for years been very angry at a man who was a real pain in the posterior finally came to the point where he realized he must forgive the man and forgave him sincerely. When he forgave him, his hemorrhoids disappeared. The body truly does react to our love or hate of others, and the reactions to love are far more positive and healthful than are the reactions to hate.

Therefore, if you are going to achieve optimal health, you are going to have to forgive those who have offended you and hurt you in the past and let dead dogs lie. You will also have to forgive yourself, and, if you are angry with God, you are going to have to forgive Him. Rather than trying to re-write *The Eternal Triangle* here, I would suggest you obtain a copy and read it carefully and prayerfully. However, one chapter in that book is very appropriate to the subject of health and should be reproduced here. The topic is love:

> *In a word, there are three things that last forever: faith, hope, and love; but the greatest of these is love.*
> —1 Corinthians 13:13 NEB

The Greek language, in which the New Testament was written, has three words translated as *love* into English. Although these three Greek words are entirely different, they are translated into the single English word. The three Greek words are *eros,* translated as sexual or physical love; *philos*, which means friendship or brotherly love; and *agape*, which means unconditional love. It is the word *agape* which is used to refer to the kind of love God has for us.

M. Scott Peck, M.D., in his book *The Road Less Traveled*, gives the best definition of love I have seen. In it he defines love as that action which is directed toward achieving maturity in the object of love. Love, then, is not a mushy type of thing; it is hard-nosed and practical, aimed at bringing another to maturity and wholeness. Marriage, which at its best brings out the best in both husband and wife, should be based upon that type of love. *Eros* and *philos* do not last; *agape* does. When a man and woman live together committed to helping the other achieve maximum potential, then that marriage will succeed. However, this is a mutual endeavor; marriage should not be entered into with an agenda for the spouse's improvement. Love exists when each makes possible and encourages maturity in the other. Maturity requires freedom to grow.

My dear friend Dr. Bruce Morgan says that the purpose of God in your life is to free you to become what He created you to be. Each of us is unique in the universe, and there will never be another like any one of us. God's will for your life is that you become who you are in Christ. That may sound like a contradiction, but those of us who have lived a few years know all too well that we tend to mask our true selves and live as hypocrites. This is more pronounced in children as they strive to please their parents and later their peers. Most of us eventually either come to be ourselves or live with internal conflicts which lead to personality disorders. Happiness is not found in living out the expectations of others; it is found in living out our own lives, if our lives have been put under the guidance of our heavenly Father.

Perhaps it would be better to say that God's will for us is that we become whom He sees us to be. If we will surrender our lives to Jesus as Lord and receive the indwelling Holy Spirit, then we become new creations. That creation has a destiny in the mind of God, and that is the person God wants to form in us. If you are still an unregenerate person, perhaps it is best for you to keep that "you" bottled up within you.

Love, in this sense, acts to secure the success and mature growth of the object of its love insofar as this action does not impede or interfere with the maturity or success of another. One can love one's enemies without liking them, because it is entirely possible to desire one's enemies success and fulfillment in life (insofar as it does no harm to others) and still not want to associate with them. The great commandment is to love the Lord our God with all our strength, mind, and heart. The second commandment is to love our neighbor as ourselves. Obviously, it does our neighbor no good to be loved as we love ourselves if we actually hate ourselves; it is assumed that a healthy person will love himself. All God asks is that we love others with equal devotion. Love, of course, being defined as acting toward the maturity of the person being loved.

> *Love is patient and kind; love is not jealous or boastful; it is not arrogant or rude. Love does not insist on its own way; it is not irritable or resentful; it does not rejoice at wrong, but rejoices in the right. Love bears all things, hopes all things, endures all things.*
> —1 Corinthians 12:4-7 RSV

The nature of God is love. Therefore, God blesses the good and wicked alike. That is why, if the love of God is indeed within us, we should bless, and not curse, our enemies. Obviously, that is not to mean that we hope they will prevail against us or that they will have success in doing evil. But we should be like our Father and pray that they be blessed in doing good. There is a difference. In the end, the best way to get rid of an enemy is to turn him into a friend and brother.

Of the scriptures, chapter 13 of First Corinthians and the entire First Letter of John seem to be the most comprehensive on the subject of love. Jesus' sermon on the mount (Matthew 5-7) defines the unconditional love of God and sets the standard by which we will be judged. Without the gift of love in our hearts, given to all who have accepted Jesus as Lord and Savior (1 John 3:1 RSV) we would never be able to live up to that standard. But through His grace God has freely given us His nature, which is love. Please notice that God's love for you is unconditional: you can be an adulterer, murderer, and a thief; He still loves you and wants the best for you. But His love is not without limits: He will leave you alone and God-forsaken if you persist in refusing to accept His forgiveness by giving your loyalty to Jesus as Lord.

If we can come to understand that God is love, and that God's will in our lives is that we receive the best in this life and achieve maturity, then we can come to trust God to deal rightly with us. The word that is translated as *salvation* carries with it the meaning of good health, prosperity, social well-being, and happiness. The Hebrew word *shalom* has the same galaxy of meaning. Love, then, acts to establish salvation in the life of the object of that love. It is an act of love to discipline a child to correct immature or bad behavior. It is equally an act of love for our heavenly Father to discipline us for our maturity, even as He disciplined Jesus to bring him to maturity. We cannot expect to be sons of God without His discipline. The term *son of God* in this context does not exclude women; it is used in the sense of legal maturity, as when a Roman child was given legal status as heir of the father's estate.

In the days of his earthly life he offered up
prayers and petitions, with loud cries and tears, to

God who was able to deliver him from the grave.
Because of his humble submission his prayer was
heard; son though he was, he learned obedience in
the school of suffering, and, once perfected, became
the source of eternal salvation for all who obey
him, named by God high priest in the succession of
Melchizedek.
—Hebrews 5:7-10 NEB

My son, do not think lightly of the Lord's dis-
cipline, nor lose heart when he corrects you; for the
Lord disciplines those whom he loves; he lays the
rod on every son whom he acknowledges.
  You must endure it as discipline: God is treating
you as sons. Can anyone be a son, who is not dis-
ciplined by his father? If you escape the discipline
which all sons share, you must be bastards and no
true sons.
—Hebrews 12:5-8 NEB

No one likes to be found lacking, nor to be disciplined.
However, discipline is not necessary for the son who
constantly seeks to walk in the will of the Father. It is far
better to seek the will of the Father in prayer and to obey
his guidance than it is to walk without that guidance and
learn by trial and error. Seeking guidance in advance is
itself a form of discipline. Self-discipline is better than
discipline imposed from above, whether from God, your
profession, or the government. That is why Paul writes
that there is no law against love.

The miracle is that love is a gift from God. Our Father does
not expect us to love others with a divine love we muster up
ourselves: He gives us this love, for without it we could not
be said to be the sons of God. This divine love instilled within
us allows us to love the unlovely, and it comes with the
indwelling Holy Spirit, for God Himself is love.

*See what love the Father has given us, that we
should be called children of God; and so we are.*
—1 John 3:1 RSV

*God is love; he who dwells in love is dwelling in
God, and God in him.*
—1 John 4:16 NEB

Thus God is not asking us to do the impossible. In His
grace He has given us the power to love by instilling His
divine love within us. For that reason we can say with
confidence that anyone who is not walking in love with
his fellow man or with other Christians is not a Christian,
for as Jesus said:

*I give you a new commandment: Love one
another; as I have loved you, you are to love one
another. If there is this love among you, then all
will know you are my disciples.*
—John 13:34-35 NEB

Do those of us who are called Christian live up to this
standard? Is there any wonder why the world does not take
us seriously when the history of the organized church is
written in blood? Yet, during it all, there have been Godly
men and women who lived the life of love set before them.
There are yet those to whom Jesus is indeed Lord. It is not
fair to judge Jesus by the lowest examples among those of
us who call ourselves Christian, but by the highest. For it
is certain to those who have studied human history that
without Jesus as our example we would still be living in
darkness and amidst terrible evil.

However, it cannot be said that the love of God is
without limits, for it is plain in scripture and human history
that God will eventually quit striving with a man or nation
which refuses to mature and walk in love. The first and

second chapters of Paul's Letter to the Romans makes that amply clear. God will give you up and let you go your own way outside His influence if you persist in rebellion. Think back on the last few weeks of your life and realize how the guidance or check of the Spirit kept you from doing something you would most certainly have regretted forever. It would be terrible to be God-forsaken. Even worse to be in rebellion against God and also to be God-forsaken. If you find yourself in a struggle with God, you are not God-forsaken, nor have you committed the unpardonable sin. God doesn't strive with those whom He has given up. But don't press your luck: God's patience has its limits.

God is love. Those who walk in love with their fellow man demonstrate within their lives the presence of God. Those who in their fervor would kill you to prove their religion neither know God nor are known by God. By their fruits their nature is shown. It is not possible to fake the love of God, nor is it possible to hide it. Like a light shining in the darkness, it cannot be hidden.

The law of love is summed up by Jesus:

So whatever you wish that men would do to you, do so to them; for this is the law and the prophets.
—Matthew 7:12 RSV

You shall love the Lord your God with all your heart, and with all your soul, and with all your mind. This is the great and first commandment. The second is like it: you shall love your neighbor as yourself. On these two commandments depend all the law and the prophets.
—Matthew 22:37-40 RSV

If you have a healthy relationship with the Father as a result of being forgiven and accepting Jesus as Lord, you should love yourself, because God loves you, and you should do no less. If you then, being loved, love your neighbor as yourself you will fulfill the "golden rule" of doing unto others as you would that they should do unto you. If you are wise, you will appreciate what great thing the Father has done for you, and love Him with all your heart, soul, and mind. Love, therefore, is the fulfilling of the law. If we allow the love that God implanted within our hearts to control our actions, then we will have earned the right to be called Christian, and to be blessed by others. Let this love be within us that was within Christ Jesus, the presence of God Himself.

Recommended Reading List

Airola, Paavo, Ph.D., N.D. *How to Get Well: A Handbook of Natural Healing.* Phoenix, AZ: Health Plus Publishers, 1974.

Becker, Robert O., M.D., and Gary Selden. *The Body Electric: Electro-magnetism and the Foundation of Life.* New York: William Morrow & Company, Inc., 1985.

Cranton, Elmer M., M.D. and Arline Brecher. *Bypassing Bypass.* Trout Dale, VA: Medex Publishers, Inc., 1990. [I recommend this as the best available book on chelation therapy (written to a layman) and on free radical pathology.]

Eccles, Sir John. *The Wonder of Being Human.* Boston: New Science Library, 1985.

Gerras, Charles, ed., with the staff of *Prevention* magazine. *The Complete Book of Vitamins.* Emmaus, PA: Rodale Press, 1977.

Kharasch, Norman, ed. *Trace Metals in Health and Disease.* New York: Raven Press, 1979.

Kunin, Richard A., M.D. *Mega-Nutrition: The New Prescription for Maximum Health, Energy, and Longevity.* New York: McGraw-Hill Book Company, 1980.

Langer, Stephen E., M.D., and James F. Scheer. *Solved: the Riddle of Illness.* New Canaan, CT: Keats Publishing,

Inc., 1984. [This book is a very thorough and readable book on hypothyroidism. I urge every physician and intelligent reader to buy and study this book. The information in it is vital to good health.]

Lovelock, Jim E. *Gaia: A New Look at Life on Earth.* Oxford: The Oxford University Press, 1979.

Lynes, Barry. *The Healing of Cancer.* Queensville, Ontario: Marcus Books, 1989.

Moore, Richard D., M.D., Ph.D., and George D. Webb, Ph.D. *The K Factor: Reversing and Preventing High Blood Pressure without Drugs.* New York: The Macmillan Publishing Company, 1986.

Ott, John N. *Light, Radiation, and You.* Old Greenwich, CT: The Devin-Adair Company, 1982.

Passwater, Richard A., and Elmer M. Cranton, M.D. *Trace Elements, Hair Analysis and Nutrition.* New Canaan, CT: Keats Publishing Company, Inc., 1983. [Highly recommended as the definitive work on hair analysis.]

Pauling, Linus, Ph.D. *Vitamin C, the Common Cold, and the Flu.* New York: W. H. Freeman, 1976.

Pearson, Durk, and Sandy Shaw. *Life Extension: A Practical Scientific Approach.* New York: Warner Books, 1982. [This book has an extensive bibliography.]

Price, Weston A., D.D.S. *Nutrition and Physical Degeneration.* Santa Monica, CA: Price-Pottenger Foundation, 1970. [This book is priceless.]

Seelig, Mildred S., M.D. *Magnesium Deficiency in the Pathogenesis of Disease.* New York: Plenum Publishing,

1980. [This is the definitive work on magnesium metabolism.]

Shute, Wilfrid E., M.D. *Health Preserver: Defining the Versatility of Vitamin E.* Emmaus, PA: Rodale Press, 1977.

Shute, Wilfrid E., M.D. *Vitamin E for Ailing and Healthy Hearts.* Pyramid, 1972.

Todd, Gary P., M.D. *Nutrition, Health, and Disease.* West Chester, PA: Whitford Press, 1985.

Yiamouyiannis, John, M.D. *Fluoride: The Aging Factor.* Health Action Press, 1986.

About the Author:

Gary Price Todd, M.D., was educated at Carson-New-man College in Tennessee and The Bowman Gray School of Medicine of Wake Forest University. As a naval officer, Dr. Todd served as a shipboard medical officer and as the Director of Hyperbaric Research at Groton, Connecticut; he then began his specialization in ophthalmology and from July 1974 to July 1977 served as Chief of Ophthalmology for the American community in Japan. Dr. Todd's wide range of interests and accomplishments have led him to be the holder of two patents and the author of several medical papers. He is also the author of *The Eternal Triangle*; *Nutrition, Health, and Disease*; and *Eye Talk*.

Dr. Todd currently practices ophthalmology in Waynesville, North Carolina, and was on the surgical staff of the Haywood County Hospital, in Clyde, North Carolina. Currently, partially paralysed from an injury, Dr. Todd no longer performs surgery.